"Freud said adolescence was a chance at a cure, one that often enough ends in complete devastation. The western world seems to be traversing a volatile adolescence, searching for a new form of maturity. Carl Waitz's book is a stunning guide for a world without any rites of passage."
Jamieson Webster, *author and psychoanalyst*

"The kids are not ok—smart and kind they may be, but anxious and over-worked; suicide second to accidents as a killer of teens. This meticulously argued and solidly researched book addresses burning questions relevant to youth mental health. Combining Lacanian psychoanalysis with sociology and anthropology, Waitz builds an indispensable clinical tool that opens new intellectual vistas."
Patricia Gherovici, *psychoanalyst and author of* Transgender Psychoanalysis

Youth Mental Health Crises and the Broken Social Link

This book critically examines the circumstances surrounding the failure of rites of passage in U.S. society and its relationship with the mental health crisis overtaking youth in America today.

The book develops a Freudian understanding of rites of initiation and the larger social link based on Freud's psychoanalytic myths read through a Lacanian lens. It further surveys the deterioration of common civil identifications in the United States, the advancement of consumer capitalism in the late 20th century, and the development of social media in the 21st century as each composing a tectonic shift destabilizing the traditional function of the rite of initiation. As a result, adolescents today have no reliable method of entering the social link through symbolic identification, nor the ability to use it to bind their libido. The book traces the clinical consequences of this failure to the recent waves of mass psychogenic illness in adolescents, the rocketing increase in psychiatric hospitalizations, and the dramatic rise in suicidal thoughts and behaviours in the past years. It also offers possible pathways forward for both adolescents and psychoanalytic clinicians working with them.

Drawing on multiple psychoanalytic schools of thought and clinical experience, this book is a vital resource for psychoanalysts, psychotherapists, and clinicians working with adolescents.

Carl Waitz, PsyD is an attending psychologist at Boston Children's Hospital and on faculty at Harvard Medical School. He supervises psychiatry and psychology trainees, teaches at Boston University, and has served as President of the Massachusetts Association for Psychoanalytic Psychology. He has a small private practice serving adolescents and young adults.

Youth Mental Health Crises and the Broken Social Link

A Freudian-Lacanian Perspective

Carl Waitz

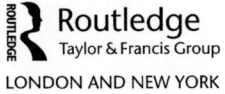

Routledge
Taylor & Francis Group

LONDON AND NEW YORK

Designed cover image: © Getty Images

First published 2025
by Routledge
4 Park Square, Milton Park, Abingdon, Oxon OX14 4RN

and by Routledge
605 Third Avenue, New York, NY 10158

Routledge is an imprint of the Taylor & Francis Group, an informa business

© 2025 Carl Waitz

British Library Cataloguing in Publication Data
A catalogue record for this book is available from the British Library

Library of Congress Cataloging-in-Publication Data
A catalog record has been requested for this book

ISBN: 9781032666327 (hbk)
ISBN: 9781032666310 (pbk)
ISBN: 9781032666334 (ebk)

DOI: 10.4324/9781032666334

Typeset in Optima
by Taylor & Francis Books

This work is dedicated to CT

Contents

PART IV
Psychoanalysis in Society

Acknowledgments

This book would not have been possible without the generous support of many people. I would first and foremost like to thank my wife, without whom I would have had neither the time nor the resolve to complete this effort. I would also like to thank my colleague Kai Bekkeli, whose readiness to discuss this work over the years of its development greatly sharpened it. I cannot recall how many of the texts I make reference to in this book were referred to me by him originally. In addition, I would like to thank Routledge for the opportunity to publish this work and to my editorial team for their patience with my pace of writing.

Introduction

This book is a response to the youth mental health crisis in the US from the perspective of Freudian-Lacanian psychoanalysis. It is a product of over a decade of working with youth in some capacity and reflects a series of interrelated ideas that are oriented toward opening discussion rather than providing definite answers.

Working in various institutions during the past ten years has probably oriented me toward the more severe range of symptomatic concerns for youth, although I have also maintained for years a private practice for outpatient care of youth. As a result of working in non-psychoanalytic institutions, my engagement with non-psychoanalytic research in this text reflects, in some ways, the sort of bridging I am used to conducting.

I believe the context of my institutional work and my attempts to bridge psychoanalytic and non-psychoanalytic thought is important, as it may seem unusual to use Freudian-Lacanian psychoanalysis in conjunction with something framed in public health terms as a "mental health crisis." Lacanian psychoanalysis does not typically concern itself with "mental health" as a construct, and there is certainly some tension in the placement of these two spheres in close proximity. However, the youth mental health crisis, measured and defined by the surveillance apparatuses of the U.S. mental health field, has an influence upon the clinic and its effects appear in the complaints and concerns of the youth that come for treatment. As a result, I believe an engagement between psychoanalysis and "mental health" is not only warranted in this case, but that psychoanalysis has something unique to offer, which will be unveiled in the course of each proceeding chapter.

As it stands, the literature on youth from a Lacanian perspective is relatively sparse in the Anglophonic world, and what there is has been, in many cases, originally written in other milieus than the US.[1] My hope is to contribute to and continue the work that has already begun by others in the US to bridge this gap,[2] in particular by addressing what has been on the mind of so many across society in recent years.

Some clarifying notes here will be instructive for reading this book. First, Lacan is notoriously difficult to read. This book is not an introduction to Lacan, but I have taken pains to try to make it accessible to those with some

DOI: 10.4324/9781032666334-1

familiarity to the field of psychoanalysis. Lacanian psychoanalysis, in my view, is characterized by a complexity that is not fully communicable in book form, yet I also believe it can be written with some degree of clarity without sacrificing too much of its essence. Whether I will be successful in the effort to make Lacanian analysis approachable without engendering excessive loss remains to be seen, and I am sure reviewers will let you know how I have done.

My use of "Freudian-Lacanian" is an intentional one. Lacan considered himself a Freudian to the end (Lacan, 1981/2011), yet his reading of Freud was revisionist sometimes setting aside some of Freud's developments and privileging others, at other times attributing meaning to Freud's words that do not quite shake out. This means that one cannot simply be Freudian if one wants to include Lacan's insights; similarly, there is no Lacan without Freud, whose work grounded Lacan, however expansive the latter's theories eventually became. My emphasis on both Freud and Lacan is meant as an admission on my part that I do not fully believe either of them. In general, Lacan's developments, and the developments of those after him, are quite compelling; I find them most compelling when connected to Freud's work. When I refer to Freudian or Lacanian ideas without compounding them, it is generally an acknowledgment that I am focusing at that time on psychoanalytic theory in the wake of one of them or the other. On a related textual note, I often refer to works by Lacan and Freud by name to ease readability (rather than rely solely upon years of publication to cue readers as to which work I am referencing).

Another note to clarify is that, although I use the structural concept of initiation rites, I am not relying on the ethnographic data that characterizes the often dehumanizing work of typically white, typically male anthropologists in the late 19th and early 20th centuries. Van Gennep (1913/2017), for his part, was somewhat better than his peers in his thoughtfulness about ethnographic data, sharply criticizing Durkheim in a notorious and scathing review for not showing adequate conscientiousness in evaluating ethnographic data. Moreover, he wrote in this review of Durkheim's (1912/1995) work:

> In ten years, his entire systematization of the Australian material will have been utterly rejected, along with the multiple generalizations constructed on the flimsiest foundation of ethnographic facts I have ever observed. The idea he has extracted from this ensemble of primitive man...and "simple" societies is simply misguided. The better one is acquainted with Australian societies, and the less one focuses on the development of their material culture and social organization, the more one remarks that they are very complex, very far from the simple or primitive, and indeed very evolved along their own lines.
>
> (Van Gennep, 1913/2017, p. 577)[3]

In this case, Van Gennep showed somewhat more circumspection and reflexive self-consciousness about how he and his peers were thinking and writing about indigenous peoples. Nonetheless, the notion of colonial Europeans and Americans extracting knowledge from a people—typically colonized people of color classed as "primitive" or "savage"—to be used for their own benefit is obviously troubling and wrong. My hope in returning to sources like Van Gennep and Durkheim is to take the ideas about which they wrote and use them constructively in a way that might benefit the diverse population of youth in the US today. However, this leads to one related challenge I must clarify, which is structuralism.

The idea that one might discern from a series of particulars a structure that is universal bears some similar problems—is there such a thing as a universal structure of the human mind? Can what a colonial white man elaborated as a structure based on ethnographic data, collected by other white men from indigenous people in a very different society, then be considered universal? I believe there are two issues at play here. The first is, again, the problematic practice of anthropology as a colonial study. Framed as above, it seems difficult to answer "yes" to the question of the universal. However, coming from another direction, not one of induction but one of deduction, the rules of language that Lacan laid out over the course of his career seem quite seriously to contend with the universality of language and the universality of its impacts on speaking beings. This is not to say that Lacan considered all languages and cultures as structurally identical; he did not.[4] But there are certain structural implications of language that Lacan spent his career exploring, just as Freud spent his career developing a metapsychology alongside his technique.

It is in the sense of looking back at the structural notion of initiation rites through a Freudian-Lacanian lens that I return to this earlier work. The return to Durkheim, in particular, is warranted by following Lacan's conception of the social link to (one of) its sources (Miller & Vaneule, 2023). Because I am not primarily interested in Van Gennep and Durkheim other than as connected to Freud and Lacan, they appear primarily in Chapter 1, with passing references throughout to connect their ideas, in an ongoing way, through each essay.

In considering the structure of the book, I should note a certain recursion the reader may observe in reading the book, particularly if read quickly. Ideas and texts come up again and again, with slight twists. Chapter 3, for example, revisits the ideas of Chapter 2, which expands on the ideas of Chapter 1. This sort of recursive writing was a decision on my part for two reasons. First, I believe the cognitive work of reading psychoanalytic texts should lay in the way one must grapple with the ideas involved—not in the pure challenge of reading unnecessarily long and complex texts. Had I avoided recursion, this would have resulted in extremely long chapters requiring a heightened commitment from the reader. The second reason for the recursive writing is that the ideas presented herein are interlocking. If I presented in Chapter 1 the discourse theory of Lacan that is presented in Chapter 5, for example, I would have missed the important scaffolding built carefully in Chapters 2, 3, and 4 to lead up to this point. Thus, if I seem to neglect a certain concept early in the book, please reserve judgment until the end—it may appear in a later chapter. If it does not, I am liable to judgment.

The book is split into four parts. In Part 1, Antecedents, the theoretical foundation for the book is laid. I attempt to highlight for those familiar with Freudian-Lacanian psychoanalysis the coordinates that I will especially rely upon; however, I also strive to make the ideas involved readable for those who are not very familiar with Freud and Lacan. I appreciate the importance that Lacanian psychoanalysts typically put on not reducing psychoanalytic concepts to simple formulations. While I'm sure there are objectionable aspects in my constructions of Freud and Lacan, I hope more advanced readers will be patient with my shortcomings in this respect as I attempted to make some complex ideas usable for novices.

In Chapter 1, the works of Durkheim, Van Gennep, Freud, and Lacan are tentatively put in conversation. Both Durkheim and Van Gennep are given some historical context, and the aspects of their ideas central to this work are connected to one another. This includes an initial foray into the definition of the social link for Lacan and sketches some initial connections between the sociological and anthropological work of Durkheim and Van Gennep and the psychoanalytic work of Freud and Lacan.

Chapter 2 elaborates Freud's various conceptions of the Father. His Oedipal father, the primal Father of *Totem and Taboo*, and the group leader of his *Group Psychology* are special areas of focus. It is the group leader in particular that I connect to Durkheim's (1897/1979) functions of integration and regulation through the identification with the ego ideal and all that this entails.

Chapter 3 revisits Freud's work from a Lacanian standpoint. In particular, Lacanian glosses on the titular aspects of social functioning in *Totem and Taboo* are considered. In presenting Lacan's work separately, I seek to make explicit the ways in which I allow Lacan to influence my view of Freud rather than to pretend they say the same thing. As Jacques-Alain Miller (2019), Lacan's son-in-law and the editor of his body of work, put it, the idea that "what Freud really said is not what Freud said" is "the inspiration of all of Lacan's teaching" (p. 110). This offers an opportunity to investigate certain obscure matters, such as how Lacan derives three different ideas— ego ideal, ideal ego, and superego—from a set of terms Freud himself cared little to differentiate.

In Part II, I address the various causes of the social link's erosion in the US from the perspective of Freudian-Lacanian psychoanalysis. This part is titled The Disease of the Infinite in reference to Durkheim's (1897/1979) reflection on desire without limits. In tracking these changes, I hope to elaborate in more detail what it is that is causing the societal changes many psychoanalysts have documented in briefer form, with particular reference to U.S. society.

In Chapter 4, I focus on the role of the leader in organizing society. This includes a brief historical survey with an emphasis on Freud's view that the Father evolved from a human man into a god and king that organized political bodies. Incorporating Robert Bellah's work on civil religion, I consider the ways in which the dissolution of such religion has implications for the integration of youth into the social link today.

Chapter 5 explores the consequences of consumer capitalism on discourse. In this chapter, I discuss Lacan's theory of discourses, including providing an interpretation of the significance of his fifth discourse, which he called the capitalist discourse. I believe the term "capitalist" in this respect is somewhat misleading from a technical standpoint; as a result, I prefer to refer to it as a consumerist discourse, as I believe it is specifically the issue of consumption that Lacan's discourse pinpoints as problematic to the social link.[5] The erosion of the prohibitive, regulatory function within the social link is a special focus here.

In Chapter 6, I consider the impact of social media and technology on youth and their entrance into the social link through initiation rites. The availability of sexual knowledge reverses the traditional relationship of child and parent in the educative process of imparting societal expectations around sex. From a psychoanalytic perspective, it is not the knowledge of sex itself that poses a problem for youth (though this certainly may be the case for some youth), but the failure of society to elaborate any particular fantasy of sexual rapport. Without such a fantasy, *jouissance* has no adequate binding in the social link.

Part III I have titled *Le Mal de la Jeunesse*, the illness of youth, in reference to Lacan's (1972) comment that perhaps this at some point might be a discourse. Although this work does not likely correspond precisely to what Lacan had in mind, it certainly takes as its reference point Lacan's reflections in the same lecture, in which he introduced the capitalist discourse. This part considers, alternately, three forms of resolution that youth have found or stumbled upon for the absence of initiation rites. What ties all three forms of resolution together is the mechanism of the purification of the pleasure ego necessitated by the capitalist discourse.

Chapter 7 considers the first of these resolutions, the least structured and most wild—the growth of suicidal thoughts and behaviors, non-suicidal self-injury, and depression among youth today. These symptoms mark less a true resolution to initiation than a very unstable, makeshift effort to bind in some way the *jouissance* that makes life unbearable when unbound.

In Chapter 8, the phenomenon of functional—that is, conversive—symptoms and the function of diagnosis-seeking in mental health care are considered as another potential, and more structured, resolution to the loss of initiation rites. By providing a symbolic nomination, such diagnostic naming categorizes one's *jouissance* within the Other, as something outside of one's control, and which simultaneously designates the proper social link, or community, for the subject based on one's diagnosis.

The final chapter of Part III, Chapter 9, considers political polarization among youth as an increasingly prominent form of solution to lack of initiation. Given the absolute privilege of the imaginary in the capitalist discourse and in the social media it has spawned, politics itself has taken on the form of a market force. By segmenting the market of the electorate according to the lines of imaginary identities, youth can find a substitute social bond in imaginary identifications that come at the cost of intolerance of difference in favor of similarity.

The book ends with Part IV, comprising a series of reflections on the role of Psychoanalysis in Society. This is especially challenging, given the increasing pressure on all organizations and communities to be active participants in the polarization of the nation. Despite the temptation to become, as a discipline or community, fully invested in political activity, these three essays make a sustained argument for the importance of psychoanalysis as something unique and different to what is already on offer in other forms of psychotherapy or social advocacy groups.

Chapter 10 considers the role of political ideology as a substitute for the surety that religion used to offer, and in particular considers whether psychoanalysis is a suitable vehicle for political ideology. This chapter presents a challenge to the use of psychoanalysis to advance specific political goals, an argument particularly important to consider in determining psychoanalysis' position with respect to the youth mental health crisis.

Chapter 11 extends the discussion of political activity by reconsidering the concept of psychoanalytic ethics. This includes an extended reflection on Lacan's (1986/1992) *Ethics of Psychoanalysis* and its significance for psychoanalytic practice today. The work of Dany Nobus (2016; 2022) is especially important in this respect.

Finally, Chapter 12 tackles the difficult question of what psychoanalysis might actually be able to offer in the context of the youth mental health crisis. I suggest two types of intervention are possible: psychoanalytically informed policy recommendations, which is an explicit deviation from psychoanalysis and inherently a risky procedure; and the elements of psychoanalytic clinical work that make it crucial in the present environment, inclusive of brief clinical vignettes to illustrate some of these points.

Overall, this book makes an ambitious attempt to connect the work of many different thinkers across nations, languages, cultures, and times to shed light on a pressing concern in the US today. There are certainly some potential objections to such an effort, which I must acknowledge at the outset. While I do not believe I have formally committed any ecological fallacies, some may easily object that the large, societal forces I consider here are not necessarily relevant to any individual youth that may enter the clinic. This is correct; it depends entirely on the singular subjectivity of the person entering the room whether the loss of initiation rites in wider society has had an effect on the youth. For example, Miller (2019) noted that those from traditionalist religions may retain the former structure of the social link;

such youth would be unlikely to experience the precise concerns outlined in this book. Nonetheless, the Internet has made the maintenance of traditional societies much more difficult in the face of the wealth of all human knowledge not only at one's fingertips, but curated by an increasingly sophisticated artificial intelligence.

Beyond the question of ecological fallacies, it is also true that the juxtaposition of many different societal forces does not in itself explain a causality. That is, just because social media has been increasingly in use, or just because political polarization is occurring, does not thereby link them to the youth mental health crisis. Technically, this is true, and I do not use data to try to argue causality from association. Rather, like others writing at the level of public health or societal trends, I utilize a theory to explain a set of data. Freudian-Lacanian psychoanalytic theory offers one possible explanation for a variety of circumstances surrounding the youth mental health crisis, and one I believe is compelling. It should be clear, however, the causal relationship is partially mediated by these theoretical constructions. Nonetheless, I am not the only one making connections between youth mental health and social media (Office of the U.S. Surgeon General, 2023), politics (Gimbrone et al., 2022), or identification with meaning-making social groups (Bamford et al., 2023), even if I am not aware of anyone combining these discussions in this way otherwise.

Finally, one other point upon which one might object is that Occam's razor would prefer to avoid the involvement of psychoanalytic theory—especially Lacan's—in explaining the problems outlined here. For example, is Lacan necessary to suggest that political polarization is bad for mental health? My answer to this is that indeed Lacan is necessary, and for two reasons. First, because Lacanian psychoanalysis problematizes what is meant by "mental health" in a way that no theory of public health does. In other words, it changes the question fundamentally to introduce Lacan. Second, the use of Lacanian theory also shifts the answer from one focused on empirical data to one centered on structural and formal concerns. Particularly in the US, there is a deep reliance upon empirical data that, while helpful in many ways, can prevent one from seeing the forest for the chlorophyll. This is an effort to refocus upon the forest by introducing something of a structural perspective. Understandably, others may not like the use of a structuralist perspective, but this seems to me to be a matter of preference and the use of different tools for different problems. In this case, I believe a structural perspective is significantly lacking in considering youth mental health and a reconsideration of structure in this context is important.

My hope is that this book will spur thinking and encourage greater engagement from those in the psychoanalytic sphere with concerns pressing on society. This is not to say I want to encourage the use of psychoanalysis for political activism, although I believe such activism is an important part of one's social (rather than psychoanalytic) role. Instead, I am hoping to encourage an engaged commentary that can bring the light of psychoanalysis to societal changes that are quite fraught and impacting those who come to treatment in ways that, whatever the singular response of the subject, provoke certain problems in subjectivity that cannot be ignored.

Notes

1 I am grateful for the translation of many projects, while still hopeful to see an increase in literature based out of the US as well. Regarding literature from other countries either written in English or translated, the work of Rodriguez (1999) in Australia, Tendlarz (1996/2003) in Argentina, and Catherine Mathelin (now Vanier; 1994/1999) in France stand out especially. The work of Françoise Dolto has also gained some attention in the Anglophonic world (see Hall et al., 2009).
2 In particular, the English language book edited by Carol Owens and Stephanie Farrelly Quinn (2017) is a wonderful collection of essays on Lacanian work with youth, and it has contributions from five psychoanalytic clinicians in the United States.
3 I am grateful for coming across this quotation in Kertzer (2019), which led me to locate the full review. Thomassen (2017) provided a helpful contextual introduction to this review from a 21st-century perspective.
4 Consider Ogasawara's (2019) reflection on Lacan's comments in this respect.
5 Holland (2015) similarly noted that the reason for calling this discourse "capitalist" is not readily apparent. His account considered the discourse as the fallout of capitalist economics, which is certainly fair; in my view, capitalism without adequate regulation results in the rampant consumerism that fundamentally takes the structure of the "capitalist" discourse. Whether such adequate regulation is possible any longer in an environment with radical technological advancement every few years is unclear and a separate question altogether.

References

Bamford, J., Leavey, G., Rosato, M., Divin, N., Breslin, G., & Corry, D. (2023). Adolescent mental well-being, religion and family activities: a cross-sectional study (Northern Ireland Schools and Wellbeing Study). *BMJ Open*, 13, e071999. doi:10.1136/bmjopen-2023-071999.

Durkheim, É. (1979). *Suicide*. G. Simpson (Ed.). (J. A. Spaulding & G. Simpson, Trans.). Free Press. (Original work published 1897.)

Durkheim, É. (1995). *The elementary forms of religious life*. (K. E. Fields, Trans.). Free Press. (Original work published 1912.)

Gimbrone, C., Bates, L. M., Prins, S. J., & Keyes, K. M. (2022). The politics of depression: Diverging trends in internalizing symptoms among US adolescents by political beliefs. *SSM - Mental Health*, 2, 100043. doi:10.1016/j.ssmmh.2021.100043.

Hall, G., Hivernel, F., & Morgan, S. (2009). *Theory and practice in child psychoanalysis: An introduction to the work of Françoise Dolto*. Routledge.

Holland, J. (2015). The capitalist uncanny. *S: Journal of the Circle for Lacanian Ideology Critique*, 8, 96–124. https://philarchive.org/archive/HOLTCU.

Kertzer, D. I. (2019). Introduction. In A. van Gennep, *The rites of passage* (2nd ed.), pp. vii–xliii. The University of Chicago Press.

Lacan, J. (1972). Du discours psychanalytique. In *Lacan in Italia 1953–1978 en Italie Lacan*, pp. 27–39. La Salamandra.

Lacan, J. (1992). *The Ethics of Psychoanalysis* (J. A. Miller, Ed., D. Porter, Trans.). W. W. Norton & Company. (Original work published 1986.)

Lacan, J. (2011). Overture to the First International Encounter of the Freudian Field, Caracas, 12 July l980. (A. R. Price, Trans.). *Hurly Burly*, 6, 17–20. (Original work published 1981.)

Mathelin, C. (1999). *Lacanian psychotherapy with children: The broken piano*. (S. Fairfield, Trans.). Other Press. (Original work published 1994.)

Miller, A. & Vanheule, S. (2023). What Holds You Together: 'The Social Link' in Durkheim, Saussure and Lacan. *Psychoanalysis and History*, 25(1), 5–29. doi:10.3366/pah.2023.0450.

Miller, J. A. (2019). *Paradigms of jouissance: Three interventions by Jacques-Alain Miller*. (T. Sowley, M. Julien, J. Haney, & A. Duncan, Trans.). Psychoanalytical Notebooks.

Nobus, D. (2016). Psychoanalytic violence: An essay on indifference in ethical matters. *Psychoanalytic Discourse*, 2, 1–20. https://psychoanalyticdiscourse.com/index.php/psyd/article/view/23/22.

Nobus, D. (2022). *Critique of psychoanalytic reason*. Routledge.

Office of the U.S. Surgeon General. (2023). *Social media and youth mental health* [White Paper]. U.S. Department of Health and Human Services. www.hhs.gov/sites/default/files/sg-youth-mental-health-social-media-advisory.pdf.

Ogasawara, S. (2019). Why Lacan says: "no one who dwells in the Japanese language has a need to be psychoanalysed". Unpublished. www.academia.edu/38073473/Why_Lacan_says_no_one_who_dwells_in_the_Japanese_language_has_a_need_to_be_psychoanalysed.

Owens, C. & Farrelly Quinn, S. (Eds.). (2017). *Lacanian psychoanalysis with babies, children, and adolescents*. Karnac.

Rodriguez, L. S. (2009). *Psychoanalysis with children: History, theory and practice*. Free Association Books.

Tendlarz, S. E. (2003). *Childhood psychosis: A Lacanian perspective*. (P. Derbyshire, Trans.). Routledge. (Original work published 1996.)

Thomassen, B. (2017). Durkheim's herbarium: Situating Arnold van Gennep's review of Émile Durkheim's The elementary forms of the religious life. *HAU: Journal of Ethnographic Theory*, 7(1), 567–575.

Van Gennep, A. (2017). Review of É. Durkheim's *Les Formes élémentaires de la vie religieuse*. (M. Carey, Trans.). *HAU: Journal of Ethnographic Theory*, 7(1), 576–578. (Original work published 1913.) doi:10.14318/hau7.1.044.

Part I
Antecedents

1 Rites of Passage and Suicide

The Youth Mental Health Crisis, Van Gennep, and Durkheim

The COVID-19 pandemic brought to public awareness something that mental health clinicians working with youth and researchers examining this population in the US already knew: A youth mental health crisis, which had been festering for many years, had reached the point of sepsis. In the decade prior to the pandemic, between 2009 and 2019, pediatric mental health hospitalizations for suicide attempts or self-injury increased by 163 percent (Arakelyan et al., 2023). Over the five years between 2016 and 2021, the latest year for which data is available from the Centers for Disease Control and Prevention (CDC), suicide has been the second leading cause of death for people between the ages of ten and 34 (Centers for Disease Control and Prevention, n.d.). The psychiatric sequelae of the restrictions imposed during the initial public health responses of countries across the world included increased psychiatric presentations of youth to emergency departments as well as increased severity of presentations (Carison et al., 2022; Khan et al., 2023). Even after the lifting of public health restrictions, some areas still saw higher rates of pediatric mental health presentations to the Emergency Department compared with pre-pandemic levels (Khan et al., 2023). In 2021 the Office of the U.S. Surgeon General released an advisory on *Protecting Youth Mental Health* that enumerated the stark depreciation in youth mental health from the late 2000s onward, noting:

> From 2009 to 2019, the proportion of high school students reporting persistent feelings of sadness or hopelessness increased by 40%; the share seriously considering attempting suicide increased by 36%; and the share creating a suicide plan increased by 44%. Between 2011 and 2015, youth psychiatric visits to emergency departments for depression, anxiety, and behavioral challenges increased by 28%. Between 2007 and 2018, suicide rates among youth ages 10–24 in the US increased by 57%. Early estimates from the National Center for Health Statistics suggest there were tragically more than 6,600 deaths by suicide among the 10–24 age group in 2020.
>
> (p. 8)

DOI: 10.4324/9781032666334-3

Later, in early 2023, the CDC released data from 2021 reflecting that nearly a third of high school females reported seriously considering suicide, and more than half of high school girls reported feeling persistent sadness or hopelessness—an endorsement 42 percent of high school student respondents made in total. In May of 2023, the U.S. Surgeon General stated that "mental health is the defining public health crisis of our time" (Cohen, 2023, para. 3). This was a bold opinion to promulgate only three years after COVID-19 brought the world to a halt, and it reflects the gravity of the real crisis facing the United States in the early 2020s.

The youth mental health crisis will raise questions for clinicians and researchers for years to come. Chief among these questions are two most crucial:

1   If the pandemic exacerbated an existing crisis, what factors contributed to the precipitation of the crisis in the first place?
2   What can be done about the crisis?

These questions are daunting and already being considered by researchers and clinicians across the country. The public health framing of the issue may especially spike the interest of epidemiologists and clinicians most deeply invested in the scalable interventions that satisfy the requirements of productivity demanded by the US's economic environment: namely, physiological interventions such as psychotropics and treatments by suggestion like behavioral medicine (see Waitz & Bekkeli, 2023). In this context, it may seem counterintuitive that psychoanalysis might have something to offer in the investigation of a public health crisis. Nevertheless, I believe to leave psychoanalysis out of this investigation would be a significant oversight on the part of anyone searching for answers to the questions the crisis raises about the psychic functioning of youth. For psychoanalysis, too, this would be a missed opportunity to engage in a clinically meaningful way with those who often dismiss its use, at least in the US. Such engagement would not constitute a form of critical social theory, which psychoanalytic writers tend to do well, but a contribution founded in the field's dedication to a unique study of the human psyche. This book is just such an engagement.

As part of the investigation into the question of what contributed to the precipitation of the crisis, there are two terms central to this book that must be considered to avoid their slippage into nothing more than academic MacGuffins—namely, *initiation rites* and the *social link*.

Regarding initiation rites, this expression finds its origin in the then-groundbreaking work of a contemporary of Sigmund Freud's, Arnold van Gennep (1909/2019), in his seminal work *Rites of Passage*. The rites of passage, as expounded by van Gennep, are the ritual practices associated with passage from one classification to another, including quite literal passages. The first form of rite of passage that van Gennep offers are the rites observed by peoples when an individual or group transitions from one physical location to another across geographical or territorial boundaries. However, Van Gennep extended the notion of a rite of passage to include transitions between social categories as well, that is, a transition from one socially constructed identity to another (e.g., impurity to purity, unmarried to married, secular to sacred, etc.).

To understand the varieties of passage he studied, Van Gennep (1909/2019) employed an essentially structural methodology to derive an understanding of their significance (in fact, his structural methodology would go on to influence the likes of Claude Lévi-Strauss, among others [Kertzer, 2019]). Van Gennep developed a structured, three-stage process at play in rites of passage. First, there is a rite of separation—some ceremony or social marking, however brief, of the separation of the novice from their current community or category. Second, the liminal rites or rites of transition mark the space between the old and new social and communal identities—not quite a member of either group, or "betwixt and between," as Victor Turner (1967, p. 93) popularized it. Third and finally, the rite of incorporation concludes the transition by establishing the identity of the novice as a member of the new community. These three stages are "not equally elaborated" or of equal length or significance in every rite of passage; Van Gennep (1909/2019) identifies rites surrounding pregnancy as primarily liminal, for example (p. 11).

The most significant portion of Van Gennep's (1909/2019) work is undoubtedly the chapter on initiation rites, which is the largest and most detailed chapter. To identify these rites as rites of *initiation* is a very specific choice of terminology, as Van Gennep critiqued other anthropologists and ethnographers for conflating puberty with initiation. In contrast, Van Gennep argued that "it is appropriate to distinguish between *physical puberty* and *social puberty*, just as we distinguish between *physical kinship* (consanguinity) and *social kinship*, between *physical maturity* and *social maturity* (majority)" (p. 68). This observation is crucial for Van Gennep, as it establishes the cultural and social structure of the transition of the novice to adulthood as an overlay upon the physiological maturation of the living organism of the human species. In other words, initiation and its attendant rites are thoroughly social constructions rather than biological processes.

Despite the disconnection between initiation and physiological maturation (particularly of sexual reproductive features), Van Gennep (1909/2019) still viewed sex as central to initiation. Initiation rites, "whose sexual nature is not to be denied and which are said to make the individual a man or woman, or fit to be one," are "rites of separation from the asexual world, and they are followed by rites of incorporation into the world of sexuality" (p. 67). For Van Gennep, this included a sorting into peer classes of the same sex, marking both an identification with the same-sex peer group as well as a regulation of sexual object choice from among the "opposite-sex" group. Obviously, such sorting is problematized today. However, the importance of this sorting process here is the way in which the initiation rite, and in particular the rite of incorporation at its conclusion, marks and permits the individual to transition into the social bond in a new and different manner, as one initiated into the secret mysteries of sexuality.

Van Gennep (1909/2019) elaborated how, in the initiation rite of separation, the novice is typically secluded from the asexual community, such as leaving the village or leaving the world of the community's children. In some cases, the novice may be symbolically killed or treated as dead. In the second, liminal rite, the novice is typically marked in some fashion. The body undergoes some procedure that results in "ineradicable traces" (p. 72), marks of identification such that one might differentiate the novice as a member of *this* group in opposition to other groups using different procedures (p. 74). Such procedures might include circumcision, tooth extraction, piercings, scarification, and so on, with Van Gennep likening the acts on the body to woodworking. Van Gennep's view is that all such body modifications are equivalent to one another as markers of *separation* from "the common mass of humanity" and serve to mark the novice as a member of a certain group, as a "sign of union" (p. 72). In the third rite, that of incorporation, the novice, if symbolically dead, is symbolically resurrected, and they are incorporated into the society of sexed adults, often receiving a new name in the process.

In Van Gennep's (1909/2019) model, there is a flow from separation from asexual childhood to incorporation in sexed adulthood, passing through a period of liminality at the end of which a new name and identity are conferred. Two corollaries follow from this model:

1   Sexual identity and sexual object choice are given meaning in socially mediated, transformative rituals, which separate biological maturation or biologically conditioned sexual qualities from the cultural and social significance overlaid upon them.
2   A change in identification–often mediated through the application of body modification–is a central component of incorporation into the community of sexed adults.

These two corollaries mark a rather ironic connection between the initiation rites that Van Gennep (1909/2019) studied and the work of his academic enemy, Émile Durkheim. Durkheim, already an eminent academic when Van Gennep began to publish in the realm of anthropology, did not take kindly to Van Gennep (1913/2017) after the latter wrote a particularly scathing review of Durkheim's (1912/1995) *Elementary Forms of Religious Life*. Primarily, he took issue with Durkheim's reliance on a few ethnographic resources to draw sweeping conclusions. This review was not the first conflict between Van Gennep and Durkheim (Thomassen, 2017), and Durkheim may have played a role in stymying Van Gennep's career (Thomassen, 2016). Despite Van Gennep's greater focus on empirical data and less ambitious theoretical inference, the two have similarities. For example, both presaged the structuralist movement in their own ways (Kertzer, 2019; Maryanski & Turner, 1991).[1]

While attempting a rapprochement between Van Gennep and Durkheim is entirely too complex for a book on youth mental health, some connection between the two must be explored. In particular, Durkheim's (1897/1979) explication of the sociological factors at play in suicide bears relevance to Van Gennep's (1909/2019) initiation rites. Durkheim (1897/1979) outlined two dimensions pertinent to suicide: integration and regulation. Integration is the degree to which an individual is incorporated into society while regulation is the degree to which society regulates the individual (its affect, opinions, behavior, and so on). Durkheim argued that these must exist in balance in order for suicide to reach its nadir.

Considering the two corollaries drawn from Van Gennep's (1909/2019) work above, one can see how the social mediation of sexuality is a form of regulation while the use of body modification or renaming to mark a change in identification is a matter of integration. This is no doubt too simple of a mapping of coordinates. For example, Durkheim's (1897/1979) theory is predicated on a reification of society as something *sui generis*. Gabriel Tarde criticized Durkheim's tendency to treat society as "exterior and superior" to the individual, as if society was some sort of "divine individual" (as cited in Niezen, 2014, p. 47) or, in Thomassen's rendering of Tarde's (1897/2000) French, a "Divine Being" (Thomassen, 2016, p. 179). Van Gennep, in contrast, did not seek to make such sweeping constructions in his work (Thomassen, 2016) and would no doubt bridle at having his work connected to Durkheim's in such a way as this. Nonetheless, the connection seems particularly important in considering the relevance of both authors for today's situation in the United States.

In fact, Durkheim's construction of society as a force independent of and greater than the sum of its individual parts is, in Michelman's (1996) view, a precursor to Jacques Lacan's development of the idea of the Other. Indeed, Michelman argues that while Lacan clearly was influenced by Durkheim, such as by citing him in his thesis on *Family Complexes* (Lacan, 1938), by the time of his seminar's recording and transcription, he no longer referenced Durkheim despite still carrying forward his influence.[2] This conceptual pedigree of the Other seems accurate, although the Other of Lacan and society for Durkheim need not be conflated. While Durkheim held that society exists and exerts influence upon its individuals, the Other of Lacan is something of an individual's (more accurately, subject's) construction—certainly represented by persons in the subject's life, but not, in the end, actually existent. In fact, Michelman contrasts Freud's and Durkheim's views on society by suggesting that Freud would see society as an avatar of the father while Durkheim would see the father as an avatar of society. Lacan arguably brings these views into synthesis, with his paternal function both connected to the Father and the Law.

The connection between Lacan and Durkheim goes further than this, however, and leads to the second term requiring exposition: the social link. In

French, the *lien social* has achieved a semantic range often lost in the Anglophonic world, where it is essentially a Lacanianism (Miller & Vanheule, 2023). Miller and Vanheule (2023) traced Lacan's use of this term to Durkheim via Saussure, arguing the work of both must be used to contextualize the idea of the social link in Lacan. Remarkably, they followed Paoletti (2004) in defining Durkheim's construction of the social link as the combination of integration and regulation, those two aspects of society Durkheim (1897/1979) discussed at length in *Suicide*, suggesting the importance of these two continua with respect to Lacan's later development of his theories of discourse, although without going on to develop this connection.[3] This relates both indirectly to the discourses as torsions of the master's discourse, but also quite directly to the degree that Lacan (1972) considered discourse to function as the social link. Indeed, Miller and Vanheule (2023) traced Durkheim's integration and regulation through Émile Benveniste's work on discourses, which they saw as influential on Lacan's later work on discourses.

The consonance—even overlap—between discourse and social link for Lacan places center stage Lacan's reliance on language in his theorization. Miller and Vaneule (2023) discussed the centrality of language in—obviously—Saussure's work as well as in Durkheim's. In Durkheim's case, they develop his employment of *representations* in his later work. They interpret his reference to the State as a privileged organizer of power as an establishment of a "privileged symbol" (p. 22). In response to this privileged symbol, the individual (in mechanical solidarity, at least) must exhibit a quantum of resemblance to the social body, which resemblance the symbol both "expresses and epitomizes...whilst simultaneously guaranteeing" (Durkheim, 1893/2014, p. 82). This privileged symbol holds "not only a repressive force that would hold contradictory representations at bay, but also a radiating energy capable of positively determining actions and shaping events" (Miller & Vanheule, 2023, p. 24). In other words, the privileged symbol retains power of both prohibition and positive injunction. Miller and Vanheule (2023) astutely relate this privileged symbol both to Freud's (1921) ego ideal as well as to Lacan's (1962) unary trait, suggesting a certain degree of affinity between their formulations.

Returning to the two stipulations of Van Gennep's (1909/2019) initiation rites—the social transmission of sexuality and the use of identification to regulate said sexuality—one can see how initiation relates to privileged symbols that govern integration (resemblance) and regulation (prohibition and injunction). In other words, the entrance into the social link as an *adult*, a class governed differently than *child*, requires the rituals of initiation that transform the novitiate from one class to the other. This is the relationship between Van Gennep's (1909/2019) rites and Durkheim's (1897/1979) social link, the one providing entree to the other, however opposite the two men may have found themselves in life.

Regarding psychoanalysis, Michelman (1996) observed that, despite being born two years apart, Durkheim and Freud had no known interaction or interchange. Durkheim never engaged with psychoanalysis, and Freud's (1913) references to Durkheim are confined to *Totem and Taboo*, wherein he considers Durkheim's views on a number of subjects related to its titular concepts. Generally, however, Freud's vision of society as originating from the psychic consequences of individuals (i.e., being born out of a group of individuals feeling guilt) is at odds with Durkheim's belief in a society, superior to the individual, that bears ontological weight. Lacan's reformulation of Freud positions him as a potential "bridge figure between Freud and the sociological tradition" (Michelman, 1996, p. 144), a point I will revisit in Chapter 5.

Despite overlapping areas of interest between sociological and anthropological ideas and psychoanalytic theory, psychoanalytic engagements with, for example, Van Gennep's (1909/2019) concept of rites of passage have been sparse. There are certainly numerous uses of the notion, in a rather truncated form, to support larger arguments (e.g., Balter, 2020; Oliveira, 2020), but these relatively unconsidered uses of the concept do not interrogate it further. Durkheim's influence on Lacan has also gone undervalued (Michelman, 1996; Miller & Vanheule, 2023). This state of things may be reflective of attempts to legitimize the psychoanalytic field in the eyes of the medical and mental health establishments, particularly in the US, where appeals to randomized clinical trials are much preferred over against interdisciplinary theoretical developments. Many non-Lacanian psychoanalysts have abandoned some of Freud's more controversial metapsychological and social ideas. In Lacanian psychoanalytic spaces, in contrast, there seems to be a mixed bag with respect to interest in interdisciplinary study. However, even where Lacanians have stuck with Freud's metapsychology, there are not many engagements with rites of passage.

The present state of psychoanalytic engagement with rites of passage notwithstanding, some psychoanalysts close to the field's inception—and a few outside the Anglophonic sphere more recently—have made attempts to engage rites of passage, particularly initiation rites as found across many societies, with psychoanalytic theory. In fact, the psychoanalytic tradition of engaging with initiation rights began with Freud's own brief remarks on initiation rites (to which I will return in the following chapter). While this chapter has briefly introduced some of the ideas of Van Gennep and Durkheim that will be relevant to the central questions of this book, the following chapters will offer greater expansion on the ideas of Freud and Lacan and their relationship to Durkheim and Van Gennep.

In light of the youth mental health crisis, one might recall that in 1972, in a characteristically peripatetic lecture, Lacan foresaw the possibility that, at some point, a discourse might emerge which could be called *le mal de la jeunesse*, the illness of youth. If there was ever a time for psychoanalysis to investigate the possibility of such a discourse, the time is now. To seek answers to a 21st-century mental health crisis in the US by returning to the theoretical elaborations of two French academics in anthropology and sociology, both born in the 19th century, may be surprising. To connect 19th- and early 20th-century conceptions of initiation rites and the social link to the state of youth in the US in the early 21st century, Lacan will indeed provide a bridge. By utilizing Freud's ideas, influenced as they were by the same milieu as Durkheim and Van Gennep, and Lacan's advancement of them over the course of his lengthy career, I hope to elaborate iteratively a series of psychoanalytic answers first to the question of what precipitated the youth mental health crisis and the second to the question of what there is to be done about the matter. Although a tall order, my hope is that these reflections will be useful at multiple levels for those working with or studying adolescents.

Notes

1 Though Durkheim's relationship to structuralism is a little more complex. See Xie (2021).
2 Lacan (1998/2017) does make at least one indirect reference to Durkheim, although this is dismissive. This is discussed further in Chapter 5.
3 Miller and Vanheule (2023) do not themselves commit to a "univocal definition of the term 'social link'" (p. 8).

References

Arakelyan, M., Freyleue, S., Avula, D., McLaren, J. L., O'Malley, A. J., & Leyenaar, J. K. (2023). Pediatric mental health hospitalizations at acute care hospitals in the US, 2009–2019. *JAMA: the Journal of the American Medical Association*, 329(12), 1000–1011. doi:10.1001/jama.2023.1992.

Balter, L. (2020). The Nicholas Young phenomenon. *IJP Open Peer Review and Debate*, 7, 1–33.

Carison, A., Babl, F. E., & O'Donnell, S. M. (2022). Increased paediatric emergency mental health and suicidality presentations during COVID-19 stay at home restrictions. *Emergency Medicine Australasia: EMA*, 34(1), 85–91. doi:10.1111/1742-6723.13901.

Centers for Disease Control and Prevention. (n.d.). WISQARS Leading Causes of Death Visualization Tool. Center for Disease Control and Prevention. https://wisqa rs.cdc.gov/lcd/?o=LCD&y1=2016&y2=2021&ct=10&cc=ALL&g=00&s=0&r=0&ry =0&e=0&ar=lcd1age&at=groups&ag=lcd1age&a1=0&a2=199.

Centers for Disease Control and Prevention. (2023). Youth Risk Behavior Survey: Data Summary and Trends Report. Department of Health and Human Services. www.cdc.gov/healthyyouth/data/yrbs/pdf/YRBS_Data-Summary-Trends_Report202 3_508.pdf.

Cohen, S. (2023, May 4). Oprah Winfrey, U.S. Surgeon General Vivek Murthy headline WOW 2023 Mental Health Summit. *UCLA Health*. www.uclahealth.org/news/oprah-winfrey-us-surgeon-general-vivek-murthy-headline-wow.

Durkheim, É. (1979). *Suicide*. G. Simpson (Ed.). (J. A. Spaulding & G. Simpson, Trans.). Free Press. (Original work published 1897.)

Durkheim, É. (1995). *The elementary forms of religious life*. (K. E. Fields, Trans.). Free Press. (Original work published 1912.)

Durkheim, É. (2014). *The division of labor in society* (W. D. Halls, Trans.). Free Press. (Original work published 1893.)

Freud, S. (1913). Totem and taboo. *The Standard Edition of the Complete Psychological Works of Sigmund Freud* (Vol. XIII, pp. vii–162). Hogarth Press.

Freud, S. (1921). Group psychology and the analysis of the ego. *The Standard Edition of the Complete Psychological Works of Sigmund Freud* (Vol. XVIII, pp. 65–144). Hogarth Press.

Khan, J. R., Hu, N., Lin, P. I., Eapen, V., Nassar, N., John, J., Curtis, J., Rimmer, M., O'Leary, F., Vernon, B., & Lingam, R. (2023). COVID-19 and pediatric mental health hospitalizations. *Pediatrics*, 151(5), e2022058948. doi:10.1542/peds.2022-058948.

Kertzer, D. I. (2019). Introduction. In A. Van Gennep, *The rites of passage* (2nd ed.), pp. vii–xliii. University of Chicago Press.

Lacan, J. (1938). *Family complexes in the formation of the individual.* (C. Gallagher, Trans.). Unpublished.

Lacan, J. (1962). Identification. (C. Gallagher, Trans.). Unpublished. www.valas.fr/IMG/pdf/THE-SEMINAR-OF-JACQUES-LACAN-IX_identification.pdf.

Lacan, J. (1972). Du discours psychanalytique. In *Lacan in Italia 1953–1978 en Italie Lacan*, pp. 27–39. La Salamandra.

Lacan, J. (2017). *Formations of the Unconscious*. J. A. Miller (Ed.). (R. Grigg, Trans.). Polity. (Original work published 1998.)

Michelman, S. (1996). Sociology before linguistics: Lacan's debt to Durkheim. In D. Pettigrew & F. Raffoul, *Disseminating Lacan* (pp. 123–150). State University of New York Press.

Miller, A. & Vanheule, S. (2023). What Holds You Together: 'The Social Link' in Durkheim, Saussure and Lacan. *Psychoanalysis and History*, 25(1), 5–29. doi:10.3366/pah.2023.0450.

Niezen, R. (2014). Gabriel Tarde's publics. *History of the Human Sciences*, 27(2), 41–59. doi:10.1177/0952695114525430.

Office of the U.S. Surgeon General. (2021). Protecting youth mental health: The U.S. Surgeon General's Advisory [White paper]. U.S. Department of Health and Human Services. www.hhs.gov/sites/default/files/surgeon-general-youth-mental-health-advisory.pdf.

Oliveira, R. (2020). The father and the paternal function in the psychoanalytical process: Theoretical and clinical issues. *American Journal of Psychoanalysis*, 80(3), 309–330.

Maryanski, A. & Turner, J. H. (1991). The offspring of functionalism: French and British structuralism. *Sociological Theory*, 9(1), 106–115. doi:10.2307/201876.

Paoletti, G. (2004). La théorie durkheimienne du lien social à l'épreuve de l'éducation morale. *Cahiers Vilfredo Pareto*, XLII-129, 275–288. doi:10.4000/ress.426.

Tarde, G. (2000). Contre Durkheim à propos de son Suicide. In M. Berlandi & M. Cherkaoui (Eds), *Le Suicide un siècle après Durkheim*, pp. 219–255. Les Presses universitaires de France. (Original work published 1897.) http://classiques.uqac.ca/classiques/tarde_gabriel/contre_durkheim/contre_durkheim.pdf.

Thomassen, B. (2016). The hidden battle that shaped the history of sociology: Arnold Van Gennep contra Émile Durkheim. *Journal of Classical Sociology: JCS*, 16(2), 173–195. doi:10.1177/1468795X15624191.

Thomassen, B. (2017). Durkheim's herbarium: Situating Arnold Van Gennep's review of Émile Durkheim's The elementary forms of the religious life. *HAU: Journal of Ethnographic Theory*, 7(1), 567–575.

Turner, V. (1967). *The Forest of symbols: Aspects of Ndembu ritual.* Cornell University Press.

Van Gennep, A. (2019). *The rites of passage* (2nd ed.), (D. I. Kertzer, Trans.). University of Chicago Press. (Original work published 1909.)

Waitz, C. & Bekkeli, K. (2023). Psychoanalytically informed care and behavioral medicine: Consideration and recommendations for evidence-based practice in institutions. *Psychoanalytic Psychology.* Advance online publication. doi:10.1037/pap0000489.

Xie, J. (2016). The structuralist twisting of Durkheimian sociology: Symbolism, moral reality, and the social subject. *Journal of Classical Sociology: JCS,* 16(1), 21–36. doi:10.1177/1468795X13497141.

2 An Oedipal Odyssey
Freud's Iterations of the Father

Freud and Initiation

The social link in Freud's work shares some consonance with Durkheim's (1897/1979) view that integration and regulation are central features of the link between the individual and society. Indeed, the social link is not simply what attaches individuals to one another but what attaches them to society or to the group. Even if Freud and Durkheim might not have seen eye-to-eye on the reification of society, they shared a sense that individuals do not simply connect directly to one another, such as through imitation—a point that Miller and Vanheule (2023) highlight. This chapter will consider Freud's social theories, particularly focusing on his views of social organization and the effects of society on the individual. Some connecting points with Van Gennep and Durkheim will be highlighted, although the primary focus is on Freudian social theory.

Freud's embrace of Darwin's (1871) primal horde for his construction of the psychoanalytic myth *Totem and Taboo* (Freud, 1913) placed the origin of the social link in what Freud considered the most fundamental law, the incest taboo. Freud envisioned the primal horde (horde, in this case, meaning something like a small familial group) as one ruled by a patriarch, the primal father (*Urvater*), who retains the females of the horde for his own sexual purposes and bars the sons from sexual enjoyment. The sons, in response, band together and murder the father. However, the ambivalent feelings of the sons toward the father lead to their regret and guilt for having killed him, and, therefore, they construct two institutions: First, the totem animal, which represents the dead father and with which the members identify, and second, the incest taboo of exogamy, the rule not to marry those within the same group, which is governed by the totem and totem clan membership. Thus, for Freud, human society is originally predicated on identification with the dead father via the totem and a renunciation of sexual promiscuity within the family or family-clan, that is, on the acceptance of the incest taboo. In this way, Freud finds the Oedipus complex at the beginning of human society; indeed, the actual Oedipal moment (the murder of the father for sexual enjoyment of the mother and sisters) is the founding act of

DOI: 10.4324/9781032666334-4

society. Just as the subject reaches the dissolution of the Oedipus complex through identification with the father and renunciation of its interest in the mother (Freud, 1924), so too did society begin with totemic identification and the taboo of the incestual object. Freud (1930) himself was explicit about the continuity between his conception of the individual's psychic formation and the formation of civilization.

With this model, Freud (1913) established that two psychical functions are involved in the foundation of the social link. The first is identification, as identification with the totem (the emblem of the dead father) is the mediating function by which the individual gains a relationship to a wider society. The second function involved is the Law, which instates the incest taboo. It is significant that the identification with the totem is intertwined with the cultural incision into sexual life of humans—the incest taboo, an incision not generally present in the animal kingdom (De Boer et al., 2021)[1]—rendering the Freudian conception of civilization as predicated on sexuality. Without facilely applying Van Gennep's (1909/2019) rites to the myth of the primal horde as if it were historical, one can nonetheless observe the structural components involved in the myth. There is a passage from asexual child to sexed adult wherein the sons place themselves at the level of the father (that is, transition from child to adult) by accomplishing his murder. There is a liminal period marked by uncertainty, guilt, and remorse—befitting Douglas's (1966) association of transitions with danger. In the end, incorporation is accomplished through identification. Moreover, one can easily see the two vectors of both Van Gennep's initiation rites and Durkheim's (1897/1979) society:

1   The regulation of sexual identity and sexual object choice in the taboo.
2   Integration into a society as governed by a privileged symbol.

Even if Durkheim and Van Gennep may have held disagreements with Freud on the exact significance of totemism, the importance of the totem for social cohesion and integration for all three is instructive here. Similarly, although taking different avenues to arrive at their destination, each also stressed the regulation of sexuality explicitly (in Freud and Van Gennep) and desire more broadly (in Durkheim).

The notion of the incest taboo as foundational to society is not as far-fetched as some might imagine; humans in the Upper Paleolithic, long before written history, seem to have engaged in sexual reproduction only with those outside of their close relatives in contrast to at least some of the now extinct Neanderthals (Sikora et al., 2017). Freud (1930) considered the renunciation of drive satisfaction, first and foremost the renunciation entailed in the incest taboo, as fundamental to civilization. He wrote at length about this in *Civilization and Its Discontents* and revisited it in *Moses and Monotheism* (Freud, 1939). The essential step taken by the children of the primal horde is Freud's colorful explanation of the more abstract principle that "human life in common is only made possible when a majority comes together which is stronger than any separate individual and which remains united against all separate individuals" (Freud, 1930, p. 95). Notably, the extent to which the majority "remains united against all separate individuals" marks a measure of agreement between Freud and Durkheim's (1897/1979) conception of an external and superior society, even if the "majority" for Freud is a collection of individuals. Furthermore, Freud (1930) described that "the members of the community restrict themselves in their possibilities of satisfaction, whereas the individual knew no such restrictions" (p. 95). For Freud, the individual trades the *possibility* of complete drive satisfaction (in reality, only available to the strongest individuals) in exchange for the safety of the group.

Freud's (1930) sensibilities echo those of Durkheim (1897/1979) 33 years before, who argued that the role of regulation is to place a limit on what would otherwise be an infinite human desire. Where Freud considered the practical limits of the drive as an especially sexual function (i.e., only the strongest could actually enjoy), Durkheim considered society as the only agency capable of directing human desire in a delimited and therefore safe fashion. Rather than marking a break between Freud and Durkheim, this seems to suggest instead that what Freud would consider the chaos of all-against-all would, from a Durkheimian perspective, already constitute a form of societal regulation (such that the strong would enact society's limitations on the weak), although the strong themselves would potentially suffer from some rudimentary form of anomie—up until the formation of the majority that would places limits across all members. Freud (1930) viewed this sort of equitable justice as the foundational principle of civilization, namely, that no one is spared from the law however strong they may be. The civilized exchange is thus that of "a portion of [one's] possibilities of happiness for a portion of security" (p. 115).

In addition to this form of societal regulation, Freud (1930) was unconvinced about the feasibility of common life unless the individual makes some libidinal investment in society. In his view, "necessity alone, the advantages of work in common, will not hold [peoples] together" (p. 122). This is because the aggressiveness resulting from the death drive would too easily overwhelm such a loose connection. Setting aside the discussion of the death drive for the moment, it seems fair to note that human history is rife with examples in which propinquity alone did not serve a protective function for neighboring peoples.

Thus, society bears a need for sublimation, for its members to transfer some of the libido that would otherwise be invested in sex and family into the group. This is the other foundation of the social link in Freud, that the individual has a finite quantity of libidinal resources to invest and chooses to invest a portion of it in society. In this way, sexuality is the cornerstone of all social ties for Freud. The libidinal investment is, of course, freed up by the prohibition of the Law against incest; the prohibition is the condition of the individual's entrance into society. This is why Freud (1930) considered the family the "germ-cell of civilization" (p. 114), as each family's law of exogamy leads to social linking in groups.

Indeed, it is at the intersection of the libidinal investment in the family and the libidinal investment in society that Freud (1930) located the tension of the rite of initiation. It is initiation rites that mark the passage from the family into the larger social link. Freud described how the family unit is loath to surrender a member to society:

> We have already perceived that one of the main endeavors of civiliza-tion is to bring people together into large unities. But the family will not give the individual up. The more closely the members of a family are attached to one another, the more often do they tend to cut themselves off from others, and the more difficult is it for them to enter into the wider circle of life. The mode of life in common which is phylogeneti-cally the older, and which is the only one that exists in childhood, will not let itself be superseded by the cultural mode of life which has been acquired later. Detaching himself from his family becomes a task that faces every young person, and society often helps him in the solution of it by means of puberty and initiation rites.
>
> (p. 103)

Freud here mixes the notion of puberty and initiation, as Van Gennep (1909/ 2019) so disliked, but it is clear Freud (1930) has in mind the cultural rather than the biological underpinnings of the transition to adulthood. In Freud's account, the parents are wont to retain the child *as their object* for as long as possible. This is, in essence, the same observation Lacan (1986/2018) makes in his "Note On the Child," wherein he warns that without the intercession of the Law, the child becomes captured as the object of the family within the family fantasy.[2] One important observation to make here is that the object within the family fantasy is not necessarily an object welcomed by the family. While the child may be a treasured object, it is no less likely— and possibly more likely—the child in this case will be the monstrous object, loved in the sense of being abhorred or hated. Regardless of the relation (loving or hating) of the family to the child-as-object, the question remains, in what way does the initiation rite help to navigate the child's passage from the family to society?

Freud identified the initiation rite most readily with circumcision, which he viewed (along with other ritual excisions and resections) as relics of cas-tration (Freud, 1933; see Freud, 1916). This is precisely in line with Van Gennep's (1909/2019) view. Freud (1938) viewed the symbolic castration accomplished in initiation rites as "an expression of submission to the father's will" (p. 190). The father's will, which is unambiguous in Freud, is the imposition of the renunciation of satisfaction in the incest taboo (Freud, 1933, pp. 86–87). The separation of the novice from other-sexed community members during rites of initiation also signifies the separation from the family involved in the process; for the male novice, separation from the mother, and for the female novice, separation from the father. Often, the same-sexed parent would participate alongside the novice (Van Gennep, 1909/2019). For Freud, the initiation rite is a symbolic entrance of the subject into the adult social link by way of submitting to the incest taboo, just as the children of Freud's primal father established the social link in this way, redirecting libidinal investment into the social link as organized by the totem.

Again, this submission to "the father's will" (Freud, 1938, p. 190) bears a striking similarity—as observed by Miller and Vanheule (2023)—to Durkheim's privileged symbol in society. With Freud's theory of libido in hand, the connection between Durkheim's integration and regulation becomes clear: the individual is capable of integration into society to the extent that it submits its desire to the regulation of society, thus freeing up libido for the investment of integration.

This structural framework of the initiation rite highlights the *separation rite* of the novice's departure from the asexual realm of children, where sexes are often intermingled, and the *incorporation rite* that inducts the novice into the realm of sexed adults, where the sexes are often separated precisely because of the sexual difference. This leads Van Gennep (1909/2019) to assert, just as Freud might, that "though [initiation rites] are independent of puberty, they are of a sexual nature, since they incorporate the boys and girls into the adult society of the sexes" (p. 86). Notably absent from this construction is the liminal rite, the rite of transition, that moves the novice from separation to incorporation. Despite noting that initiation rites might privilege rites of transition (p. 11), Van Gennep identifies body modification in initiation as "a rite of separation…which automatically incorporates [the novice] into a defined group" (p. 72). In other words, one of the most frequently cited elements of initiation for Van Gennep is most closely tied to the preliminal separation and postliminal incorporation rites; however, he does also grant that "sometimes the initiation takes place all at once, and sometimes in stages" and that in some cases, ritual periods (e.g., symbolic death) would last "for a fairly long time" (p. 75). In a Freudian accounting, separation and incorporation are doubtlessly the most important elements of entry into the social link, however much time one spends in liminal periods notwithstanding.

Further Fathers

The Oedipus complex and the myth of *Totem and Taboo* are self-similar fractals, each corresponding to the other at different levels in Freud's view; "as above, so below; as below, so above" (Three Initiates, 1912, p. 113). This unfolding symmetry suggests the investigation of the individual's psychic structure may have yet more to yield in understanding the social link.

For example, Freud (1921) extended his consideration of the totemic identificatory process in his *Group Psychology and the Analysis of the Ego*. Freud considered the group to be a "revival of the primal horde" (p. 123) and the leader a recapitulation of the primal father (who, as an individual, would have a psychology attendant to such a person). Freud argued that the role of the leader in groups is essentially hypnotic, that is, the leader governs the group member's ego in place of the ego ideal, fulfilling the same role as the hypnotist. In this way, one group leader serves, via transference, as the ego ideal for each individual in a group of people, a sort of psychological parallel to the political concept of personal union.

Freud (1921) observed three forms of identification in his work on group psychology, and the first two operate similarly: identification in place of object-choice (that is, identification with the loved object) or identification with the not-loved object (that is, identifying in a jealous manner with the object one wishes *to be* with respect to the loved object). In both cases, the identification occurs with respect to a single trait, or *einziger Zug*. Freud gives a cough (e.g., a parent's cough) as an example of what might be taken as a singular trait. The third case of identification is also based upon a single point of reference (although not the *einziger Zug*). In this case, the ego puts itself in the situation of another ego, although without direct relation to that ego. Freud's example in this case is that of a girl at boarding school who receives a letter from her secret love that causes her to have "a fit of hysterics," which then spreads to other girls by virtue of their wish to analogously have such a secret lover (p. 107). Freud's distinction between this third form of identification and the others (identification with the loved or not-loved object) is apparently that the person with whom one identifies in the third form is "not an object of the sexual [drive]" (p. 108). With the first two, the psychic bond happens with either the subject or the object of the ego, that is, the organization has to do with *being* the one with whom there is a libidinal charge (subjective) or *having* the one with whom there is a libidinal charge (objective). In contrast, the third form of identification is not about being or having the object but about occupying a certain position within a psychic constellation or situation.

Freud (1921) hypothesized that in groups, each member is bound to the leader through an identification with the loved object in the ego ideal while bound to each other through identification with a common quality in the ego, which Freud supposed was the initial tie to the leader. This would make the social bond—at least in the sorts of structured groups Freud considered–essentially coterminous with the tie to the leader; if there is no tie to the leader, there is no tie between members.

Freud's (1921) formulations in *Group Psychology* are consistent with the broader context of his other writings, in which one can again see the prominent place he gives the father as a singular figure: the *Urvater* in *Totem*, the father in the Oedipus, God in *Future of an Illusion* (Freud, 1927), the leader of the group, and the man Moses (Freud, 1939). While the *Urvater* is beyond the Law, he is no less he from whom the Law issues, both in his prohibition of sexual enjoyment for anyone but himself and in the fact that his death brings about the incest taboo. Similarly, the father of the family unit, in Freud's formulation, is the center of the Law, who prohibits the child from using the mother as an insurment of enjoyment. The leader of the group, in contrast, is not defined by its function with respect to prohibition *per se*, but in its role as a usurpation of the ego ideal, in other words, replacing the individual's conscience, a form of integration. Thus, where the *Urvater* and father are connected to the prohibitive Law, the leader's role is more open-ended. Its main function is the maintenance of the group's integration, and the moral regulation it imparts in the form of cultural values is secondary to this.

The relationship between the *Urvater*, nuclear father, and leader is crucial to the Freudian conception of the social link as well as a psychoanalytic understanding of the initiation rite. The *Urvater*'s role is a construction that manages to simultaneously communicate two central elements of human social fabric: a symbol around which society coheres and the regulation of enjoyment. The initial scene of the primal father's plenary enjoyment of all women highlights the social order seen in animal communities, where powerful males (whether one or a small group) use violence to subdue and exclude other males from breeding, such as in a pride of lions (Packer & Pusey, 1982). Freud's (1913; 1930) supposition is that the specifically human element—that which separates humanity from animality—is the development of a system of regulation of enjoyment by an exchange of every individual's unrestricted use of power for restricted use of power in order to secure social stability. The myth of the *Urvater* (and more precisely, his murder) is a construction that establishes this exchange as the base of the social foundation, including the inherently sexual nature of its origins. It is an etiological myth that, in Freud's view, accounts for a phenomenon seen throughout human culture: the surrender of individual liberty for group security in a symbolic manner (i.e., through formal laws).

In turn, the father's role in the Oedipus complex is constructed to explain the transmission of the social order to a given individual; how is the regulation of enjoyment passed on to new generations? Freud (1913) first rather weakly suggested the rituals related to the father (containing the repressed events of the primal family) are transmitted from one generation to the next and are understood by following generations at an unconscious level. Later, Freud (1939) came to the much bolder conclusion that some "archaic heritage" is passed down generationally at the level of animal biology (p. 101), a sort of innate repressed knowledge that affects every human. Freud arrived at this surprisingly Jungian (and unsurprisingly Lamarckian) notion of transmission seemingly out of a sense that other methods of explanation were not satisfactory. Part of the reason this is surprising is that Freud also recognized at other moments the way that society structures the individual's psyche outside of the appeal to constitutional factors. For example, Freud (1927) recognized in religion a social structure that is distributed to the individual "ready-made" (p. 21), and that religion as a social structure provides the individual a neurosis capable of preventing the development of a private or individual neurosis. A few years before this, he also discussed the necessity of there being a method of group psychology transforming individual psychology, concluding that such transformations must happen when group members become leaders, for example (Freud, 1921).

Taking this all into account, the most credible explanation remains Freud's initial position in *Totem and Taboo*, which appears mostly satisfactory. The rituals pertaining to the father, passed down in any given society, maintain the father's position. This is slightly different from Freud's more specific position that mnemic traces of an actual archaic event (in actuality, repeated and numerous events) were passed down unconsciously. A sharper focus, and one with fewer intractable appeals to a Lamarckian biology-of-the-gaps, would be to note that what is transmitted is not a mnemic trace, but the social structure itself, through initiation rites that perpetuate it. This social structure is not the patriarchal power structure in particular, but power structure broadly, wherein there is always tension between the leader and the group (and hence the necessity of equal love from the leader to the members). This power structure has historically repeated across time and generally followed a pattern that, when abstracted from any historical substrate, reveals the structure of the fantasy of the primal family. The Oedipus complex is a microcosmic manifestation of this fantasy at an individual level, but it is no less a matter of society. As Freud (1931) characterized it, the dissolution of the Oedipus complex "initiates all the processes that are designed to make the individual find a place in the cultural community" (p. 229). In this way, the father of the Oedipus—as constructed in the individual's fantasy—transmits the elements necessary for initiation to occur at a later time, and the rituals involved therein continue the link to that privileged symbol that governs integration and regulation. This is, incidentally, Theodor Reik's (1915/1946) conclusion regarding initiation rites as well.

Finally, regarding the group leader, Freud (1921) directly connected the leader to the *Urvater* as well: "The leader of the group is still the dreaded primal father" (p. 127). More than this, "the group still wishes to be governed by unrestricted force; it has an extreme passion for authority; in Le Bon's phrase, it has a thirst for obedience" (p. 127). Where the *Urvater* is Freud's construction of the origin of society, the Oedipus' perpetual reinvigoration of the dynamics at play in the primal horde means that at the aggregate level of groups, the same themes again come into play. Notably, the identification with the father that serves a protective function at the dissolution of the Oedipus complex may come to serve a similar role in groups, that if a member is integrated enough into the group, and into the leader's graces, some suffering may therefore be avoided.

Thus, for Freud, the structure of the ego agency that pertains to social governance is established in the combination of heritage and ritual. Freud

(1927) referred to this agency at one point as the superego but which we can call, for greater precision, by the term which Freud (1921) used in relation to the group leader: the ego ideal.[3] It is the power of this ego ideal to govern social identification and regulate the drive. Without this regulation, the body would undergo what Freud called *Unlust*, or unpleasure. This *Unlust*, which is that toward which the drive pushes, is experienced consciously as unpleasure and unconsciously as enjoyment, as the body experiences an enjoyment at odds with the Law.[4] Thus, the social link is the binding of the drive through the sublimation imposed upon those initiated into adult society. During puberty, the repressed undergoes a surge upward into consciousness, owing to the strengthening of drive (Freud, 1938; 1939), and the initiation rite provides a structure and social regulation of the sublimative process. Regardless of whether it arrives before or after puberty, the foreknowledge the novice has of the initiation will provide a limit on the drive, as the novice will recognize it is forthcoming.

The interweaving of these strands of Freudian theory are not coincidental. Obviously, one part belongs to Freud's own fascination with fatherhood. Freud (1913) quite early observed that, from his vantage point, "the beginnings of religion, morals, society and art converge in the Oedipus complex" (p. 156). This fascination is what led Lacan (1966/2006) to suggest Freud's work could be boiled down to a singular question: "What is a Father?" (p. 688).

Freud's iterative development of his breathtakingly sweeping answer to this simple question is condensable to, in brief: A Father is that which provides identification and regulation. The Freudian account of the initiation rite is one in which the novice undergoes a symbolic marking which transitions them from the realm of sexless children to the realm of sexed adults by the introduction of a social knowledge of sexuality (i.e., who is allowed for whom), complete with the exogamous implications thereof. In short, the totemic identification with the ego ideal, which provides a tribelike identity, and the incest taboo, which delivers knowledge about sexual enjoyment as well as regulation of such enjoyment, are the two key moments that bring the novice from the world of childhood into social adulthood.

Initiation rites have not figured prominently in psychoanalytic literature since Freud's brief construction of the role they play in society. Nonetheless, Reik (1915/1946) carried forward Freud's work on initiation rites in a paper Freud himself found pleasing enough to award the *Imago* prize (Freud, 1918; 1919). This paper, rather than making an extensive contribution to the psychoanalytic theory of initiation rites, largely carries Freud's brief theoretical construction over into the realm of application, reviewing the initiation rites of different peoples from the angle of Freud's elaboration. Géza Róheim (1942) made similar practical contributions from his own field notes without substantively altering the larger theoretical construct. One important point both analysts address, however, is the identification of the novice with the totem-father (Reik, 1915/1946; Róheim, 1922), a point largely latent in

Freud's short considerations, although consistent with his writings more broadly. In the decades following Reik's and Róheim's contributions, much of the literature made use of the concept of initiation or "puberty" rites only insofar as either Reik or Róheim developed it This is both a testament to their enduring contribution and an indication of the lack of innovative work in this area within psychoanalysis.

Nevertheless, there are a few Brazilian authors in recent years working on initiation in the wake not only of Freud but also of Lacan. Because of the important ways that Lacan revisited and repurposed Freud's expositions, it is crucial to consider Lacan's contributions to the Freudian project prior to considering these latter-day papers on initiation rites in modern society.

Notes

1 The discussion in De Boer et al.'s (2021) meta-analysis also suggests humans do not engage in kin-avoidance behaviors based on the underlying studies reviewed. However, those studies are based upon research showing participants images either manipulated to resemble the participant or not having been manipulated to resemble the participant. The attractiveness of the image to the participant was then measured, with attraction to resemblant images considered analogous to incestuous attraction. There are obvious limitations with this model, which is not the fault of De Boer et al., but the model fails to take into account the highly personal nature (i.e., pertaining to specific persons) of incestual attraction in humans as well as the confounding role of narcissistic identifications in such an operationalization of incestual attraction.
2 Lacan (1986/2018), of course, referred to "the functions of the mother and the father" in this note (p. 1). Nonetheless, based on Lacan's development of the notion of the paternal function, it is safe to locate this outside of the immediate body of the person of the father or father-figure as the function is broader than an individual, even if embodied by one. Similarly, the "mother" may or may not be a mother or an individual person.
3 This distinction will be taken up in more detail in Chapter 3.
4 This is a Lacanian reading of Freud, admittedly. I will revisit Lacan in the next chapter, but a more complete discussion of the evolution of drives in Freud would talk an inordinate amount of time in comparison to the overall project here. In brief, however, I will note that this formulation is predicated on Lacan's interpretation of the drive as essentially a death drive, building on Freud's later developments.

References

de Boer, R. A., Vega-Trejo, R., Kotrschal, A., & Fitzpatrick, J. L. (2021). Meta-analytic evidence that animals rarely avoid inbreeding. *Nature Ecology & Evolution*, 5(7), 949–964. doi:10.1038/s41559-021-01453-9.

Darwin, C. (1871). *The descent of man and selection in relation to sex* (Vol. II). John Murray.

Douglas, M. (1966). *Purity and danger*. Routledge.

Durkheim, É. (1979). *Suicide*. G. Simpson (Ed.). (J. A. Spaulding & G. Simpson, Trans.). Free Press. (Original work published 1897.)

Freud, S. (1913). Totem and taboo. *The Standard Edition of the Complete Psychological Works of Sigmund Freud* (Vol. XIII), pp. vii–162). Hogarth Press.

Freud, S. (1916). Introductory lectures on psycho-analysis. *The Standard Edition of the Complete Psychological Works of Sigmund Freud* (Vol. XV), pp. 1–240. Hogarth Press.

Freud, S. (1918). Letter from Sigmund Freud to Sándor Ferenczi, December 3, 1918. *The Correspondence of Sigmund Freud and Sándor Ferenczi, Vol. 2, 1914–1919*, 26, 316–317.

Freud, S. (1919). Letter from Freud to Ludwig Binswanger, January 2, 1919. *The Sigmund Freud-Ludwig Binswanger Correspondence 1908–1938*, 50, 143–144.

Freud, S. (1921). Group psychology and the analysis of the ego. *The Standard Edition of the Complete Psychological Works of Sigmund Freud* (Vol. XVIII), pp. 65–144. Hogarth Press.

Freud, S. (1924). The dissolution of the Oedipus complex. *The Standard Edition of the Complete Psychological Works of Sigmund Freud* (Vol. XIX), pp. 171–180. Hogarth Press.

Freud, S. (1927). The future of an illusion. *The Standard Edition of the Complete Psychological Works of Sigmund Freud* (Vol. XXI), pp. 1–56. Hogarth Press.

Freud, S. (1930). Civilization and its discontents. *The Standard Edition of the Complete Psychological Works of Sigmund Freud* (Vol. XXI), pp. 57–146. Hogarth Press.

Freud, S. (1931). Female sexuality. *The Standard Edition of the Complete Psychological Works of Sigmund Freud* (Vol. XXI), pp. 221–244. Hogarth Press.

Freud, S. (1933). New introductory lectures on psycho-analysis. *The Standard Edition of the Complete Psychological Works of Sigmund Freud* (Vol. XXII), pp. 1–182. Hogarth Press.

Freud, S. (1938). An outline of psycho-analysis. *The Standard Edition of the Complete Psychological Works of Sigmund Freud* (Vol. XXIII), pp. 139–208. Hogarth Press.

Freud, S. (1939). Moses and monotheism: Three essays. *The Standard Edition of the Complete Psychological Works of Sigmund Freud* (Vol. XXIII), pp. 1–138. Hogarth Press.

Lacan, J. (2006). *Écrits*. (B. Fink, Trans.). W.W. Norton & Co. (Original work published 1966.)

Lacan, J. (2018). Note on the child. (R. Grigg, Trans.). *The Lacanian Review*, 4, 13–14. (Original work published 1986) https://lacancircle.com.au/wp-content/uploads/2018/04/Note-on-the-Child.pdf.

Miller, A. & Vanheule, S. (2023). What Holds You Together: 'The Social Link' in Durkheim, Saussure and Lacan. *Psychoanalysis and History*, 25(1), 5–29. doi:10.3366/pah.2023.0450.

Packer, C. & Pusey, A. E. (1982). Cooperation and competition within coalitions of male lions: kin selection or game theory? *Nature (London)*, 296(5859), 740–742. doi:10.1038/296740a0.

Paoletti, G. (2004). La théorie durkheimienne du lien social à l'épreuve de l'éducation morale. *Cahiers Vilfredo Pareto, XLII-129*, 275–288. doi:10.4000/ress.426.

Reik, T. (1946). The puberty rites of savages: Some parallels between the mental life of savages and neurotics, (D. Bryan, Trans.). In *Ritual*. International Universities Press, Inc. (Original work published 1915.)

Róheim, G. (1922). Ethnology and folk-psychology. *International Journal of Psycho-analysis*, 3, 189–192.

Róheim, G. (1942). Transition rites. *Psychoanalytic Quarterly*, 11, 336–374.

Sikora, M., Seguin-Orlando, A., Sousa, V. C., Albrechtsen, A., Korneliussen, T., Ko, A., Rasmussen, S., Dupanloup, I., Nigst, P. R., Bosch, M. D., Renaud, G., Allentoft, M. E., Margaryan, A., Vasilyev, S. V., Veselovskaya, E. V., Borutskaya, S. B., Deviese, T., Comeskey, D., Higham, T., … Willerslev, E. (2017). Ancient genomes show social and reproductive behavior of early Upper Paleolithic foragers. *Science (American Association for the Advancement of Science)*, 358(6363), 659–662. doi:10.1126/science.aao1807.

Three Initiates. (1912). *The kybalion*. The Yogi Publication Society.

Van Gennep, A. (2019). *The rites of passage* (2nd ed.), (D. I. Kertzer, Trans.). University of Chicago Press. (Original work published 1909.)

3 Lacanian Revisions of Freudian Positions

The Man Lacan

Despite the fallowing of initiation rites in psychoanalytic literature, developments of the Freudian conception of the father have nonetheless advanced. While some schools of psychoanalysis went on to focus on the mother-child dyad or upon adaptation of the ego to reality, psychoanalysis in France came to be dominated, at least for a period, by the psychoanalyst Jacques Lacan. He was as controversial a figure in his own time as he remains today. He was removed from the International Psychoanalytic Association (IPA) when he resigned from the French component society, following his colleagues, owing to conflict regarding the training process—though without realizing, any of them, that this meant their departure from the IPA (Roudinesco, 1993/1997). He and several others founded a new professional body, the *Société Française de Psychoanalyse* (SFP), a group that immediately began negotiating with the IPA for recognition as a component society. These negotiations lasted for 10 years. One particular problem was Lacan's practice of variable length sessions, something he began to publicly deny doing despite his continued use of the practice after early 1953. The IPA would never accept such violations of psychoanalytic standards. In 1963, the SFP submitted to the IPA's requirement that, in exchange for recognition, the SFP strip Lacan of his role as a training analyst. Lacan bore anger over this for some time, likening it to an "excommunication" not unlike the *herem* born by Spinoza (Lacan, 1973/1978, p. 3).

The turbulence of his professional standing withal, Lacan became well known for the yearly seminar he led from 1951 to 1980, with the seminar becoming public in 1953, the latter 27 years being transcribed and still in the process of being formally revised and published. His writings, which are smaller in volume than his lectures, still occupy hundreds of pages across multiple books. The tenor of his teaching and view of psychoanalysis has often been condensed into what he called a "return to Freud" (Lacan, 1966/2006, p. 306), seeking to correct for what he considered the deviations of theory and technique present in other schools of analysis. His teaching featured returns to many of Freud's ideas with alternate

DOI: 10.4324/9781032666334-5

interpretations, incorporating influences from Saussure, Levi-Strauss, and—as noted in Chapter 1—Durkheim, among many, many others. His frequent engagement with other disciplines has borne fruit in the fact that his works are still prominent in critical theory, literary and film criticism, and philosophy.

Lacan's style of teaching and writing gained him notoriety as an esoteric teacher and one of the most challenging psychoanalytic authors to interpret. Nevertheless, his work has found consistent support from psychoanalytic communities across the Continent and in Latin America, and his work has become increasingly prominent in the US, not only in the humanities but in clinical work as well.

To further develop the connecting points between Freud's individualist conception of group psychology (including his views of the social link and initiation) and those in the work of Durkheim and Van Gennep—and to connect all of these to the present-day situation in the US—a recursive consideration of Freudian teaching from a Lacanian perspective is necessary. As a result, this chapter will revisit the two, broad Freudian themes developed so far—totem and taboo—with a Lacanian twist.

Totem

One of the most intriguing lexical shifts over the course of Freud's career is his rather slippery use of three terms related to the ego and its functioning: ideal ego, ego ideal, and superego. This inconsistent terminology left many psychoanalysts in the position of privileging the last of these terms—superego—over the others, which Freud himself did over the course of his career. However, a closer study of these terms will be helpful in situating Lacan's reconsideration of definitions unique to each term.

In *On Narcissism*, Freud (1914) introduced the concept of the ego ideal (used, with apparent indifference, alongside *ideal ego*) to be a formation of the ego created subsequent to the withdrawal of ego-libido from the ego in childhood. This withdrawal is a result of infantile narcissism bumping up against the "admonitions of others" and "the awakening of [one's] own critical judgment" in light of "cultural and ethical ideas," that is, of the social structure that is initially transmitted by the parents (pp. 93–94). The ego ideal, in this formulation, is used as a reference by a putative and unnamed agency that enforces the ideal within the ego. It is this putative agency that is at the heart of feelings of having one's thoughts or actions observed. The reason for the creation of and libidinal investment in the ego ideal is the ego's effort to recoup the satisfaction of perfection found originally in the infantile ego prior to the civilizing influences of the family and language. In the first period, the ego is self-satisfied with its perfection, but when civilizing influence from the parents and others begins, the ego is wounded, and satisfaction is dissipated. The ego ideal is an effort at saving satisfaction by investing in an ideal version of the ego that conforms to the expectations of the parents and, consequently, society as represented by the parents. In other words, the ideal here is an ideal version of the child.

In 1915 (although not published until 1917), Freud completed *Mourning and Melancholia*, wherein he described how a part of the ego could be set "over against the other" part, exercising critical faculties on the other part (p. 247). Freud was more tentative here, not using any terms like ideal ego or ego ideal, nor did he refer to any separate partner agency that would enforce such an ideal. In this case, the creation of this part of the ego is the result of an exchange of an object cathexis for an identification when the object is lost (e.g., when a death occurs). Although describing melancholia in particular, Freud noted that the presence of this "split off" part of the ego in other psychic situations "will be confirmed by every further observation," suggesting a more integral role for this agency in the psyche (p. 247).

However, in 1917, Freud's *Introductory Lectures* revisit the same configuration found in *On Narcissism*, including the separate enforcing agency, although he used only the expression "ideal ego" without reference to the ego ideal, suggesting the degree of interchangeability Freud saw in these terms (p. 429).

Shortly after this, in 1921, the ego ideal was the subject of theoretical revisions in Freud's *Group Psychology*, wherein the ego ideal is mentioned without any putative partner agency that enforces it; the ego ideal itself is the seat of "self-observation, the moral conscience, the censorship of dreams, and the chief influence in repression" (p. 110). The ego ideal here is not only a split off part of the ego, but more importantly, the ego ideal may be superseded by the introjection of a loved object or by the hypnotist in the process of suggestion. Most crucially for this paper, however, is Freud's observation that in groups,[1] "a number of individuals who have put one and the same object in the place of their ego ideal and have consequently identified themselves with one another in their ego" (p. 116). In this formulation, the ego ideal is not only the effective conscience of the individual, but also the point of access to participation in most forms of group life or social interaction.

In 1923, Freud's *The Ego and the Id* introduced a significant further revision in the conception of the ego ideal. Here, he used the term ego ideal to connect the concept with its past iterations, but he also introduced the term *superego* for the first time as an interchangeable name for the same agency, and it is obviously this term he would go on to favor. In this more full account, Freud attempted to work through several of the disparate ideas he developed in the decade prior. There is no partner agency for the superego at this stage, consistent with *Group Psychology* and *Mourning and Melancholia*. The establishment of the agency by means of a transition from object-cathexis to identification at the loss of the object (as in *Mourning and Melancholia*) is affirmed; however, Freud also acknowledged that the first establishment of this agency during the time of the Oedipus complex is not actually related to object loss. Rather, the initial establishment of the ego ideal is in the identification with the father, which begins even before the dissolution of the Oedipus. Freud hedged on this, noting that "parents" might be a safer notion than "father" alone (p. 31 footnote 1), and subsequently also acknowledged that identification with the father is also paired with identification with the mother and that the combination of these is reflective of the degree of masculinity or femininity the subject develops in the post-Oedipal period. At this moment of Freud's work, the superego retains a very close relationship with the parents, and especially with the father, marking again the connecting point through which societal influences are transmitted to the child.

The ego ideal makes one more significant appearance in Freud's work in 1933, in his closet drama, the *New Introductory Lectures*. In these writings, Freud appears to present something akin to his original comments in *On Narcissism*, stating that the superego is:

> the vehicle of the ego ideal by which the ego measures itself, which it emulates, and whose demand for ever greater perfection it strives to fulfill. There is no doubt that this ego ideal is the precipitate of the old picture of the parents, the expression of admiration for the perfection which the child then attributed to them.
>
> (pp. 64–65)

In this account, the partnering of agencies reappears, although in this case it seems the ego ideal's silent partner is, in fact, the superego as a separate agency. However, in contrast to *On Narcissism*, wherein the ego ideal represents a perfection of the subject's ego, Freud here shifted the archaic narcissistic perfection from the child to the child's view of the parents. In this latter version, the ego ideal is an "expression of admiration" for parental perfection.

With this brief genealogy of ego ideal, ideal ego, and superego, one can begin to make sense of Lacan's segmentation of these terms into meaningfully distinct ideas, repurposing the terms to give a fuller form to that which Freud himself had difficulty articulating.

Lacan elaborated his fundamental distinctions between these three terms relatively early in his career, beginning with distinctions between the ego ideal and superego in his work on *Family Complexes* in 1938. In this early account, Lacan primarily distinguishes the two agencies by dividing the roles of repression and sublimation, the superego governing the former and the ego ideal governing the latter. The societal import of sublimation—as discussed, for example, in *Civilization and Its Discontents* (Freud, 1930)— makes a remarkable point of connection between the Durkheimian (1897/ 1979) concepts of regulation and integration and Van Gannep's (1909/2019) initiation, with repression regulating the sexual object choice of the subject and sublimation governing societal integration as a sexed being.

Subsequently, however, Lacan distinguished the ego ideal from the ideal ego on another basis. Lacan's conception of the ideal ego is predicated on his proposed Mirror Stage, described in his 1949 address in Zurich (Lacan, 1966/2006), which is the period in which the infant comes to adopt the specular image (the mirror image) as the basis of the ego itself. This is a fundamental misrecognition at the level of the *imaginary*, that is, the realm of images. The imaginary identification with the mirror image, or with the other who appears to be oneself (the mirror, the reflection in the parent's eye, the other child—these are all specular images), is the basis of the original narcissistic investment, that perfection of the child that Freud (1914) first attributed to the ego ideal but which Lacan pulled apart as the separate agency of the ideal ego. Indeed, Lacan (1966/2006; 1998/2017) insisted that Freud did not accidentally slide between these terms in his paper *On Narcissism*, and this distinction is the conclusion Lacan drew from it. The ideal ego, for Lacan, is the image of the child that could satisfy the mother's demands, the image of the child that the primary (in the sense of first) parent projects as their own object. The child's identification with this object in an uncomplicated way is the basis of many problems in childhood, as the child becomes assumed as the parental object and taken up into the parental fantasy (Lacan, 1986/2018). This is something beyond simple attempts to please the parent. Because the maternal Other[2] holds the power of life and death (to feed or not to feed), the demands the Other makes hold grave import for the child.

Because not all of the subject is included in the mirror image—in a literal sense, one cannot see the back or sides of one's body, for example—the identification with the specular image is a moment of alienation (Fink, 1995). The subject becomes a split subject, represented by Lacan with the barred S—$\bar{S}$—the bar indicating the primal repression that breaks the subject into the ego and the subject of the unconscious. The "little other" with which one identifies in the ideal ego is represented by Lacan with a *petite a* or little *a*, the *a* being the initial of the French *autre* or other. This object *a* mediates the maternal Other's desire; when the subject identifies with the ideal ego it is in an effort to be that satisfactory object desired by the Other.

In contrast to this ideal ego, Lacan (1975/1991; 1998/2017) established the ego ideal as an inherently *symbolic* agency, the symbolic having to do with the realm of abstract signification and representation and, therefore, the social. This symbolic agency is derived not from maternal demand, but from paternal desire. That is, the mother's desire of the father leads to her absence (to be with the father) and develops within her discourse a role for the father as an Other with the ability to preclude the child from being the one that satisfies the maternal Other. This, for Lacan, is castration–the distance established between the ideal ego and the subject.[3] When the object *a* therefore falls out of the ideal ego, the child is left in the position of adopting the object *a* as its own object of desire (Lacan, 1973/1978), an echo of the Freudian notion of identifying with the loved-object (in Lacan's language, the Other). This moment is one of *separation*, which separates the subject from the object and propels desire forward as the desire of the Other.

The fundamental lack of the subject with respect to the object caused by the paternal Other renders lack as the central feature of subjectivity for Lacan (1966/2006). Indeed, in Lacan's continued development of Freud's ideas, the paternal Other is increasingly associated with the infant's entrance into language, wherein symbolic language itself engenders lack by the very fact that words only come to represent things which are absent. One primary point of reference for Lacan in this respect is Freud's (1920) discussion of the *Fort/Da* game, wherein his grandson came to represent the absence of his mother in a simple game of throwing a toy and pulling it back by its string. This primordial form of language reflects the way in which the absence of the mother described above is in fact concomitant with the introduction of symbols to represent this absent mother. Because of this linguistic formulation of castration, the object the subject desires was always already lost, having existed only in the imaginary time before the child's entrance into language (Lacan, 1966/2006).

The importance of the symbolic for Lacan (1998/2017) in the moments of the ego's formation is described in exquisite detail in the year of his seminar dedicated to *The Formations of the Unconscious*. In this year of his seminar, in which he began to elaborate his graph of desire, he explored extensively the dialectic that animated this period of his teaching. The dialectic is represented in roughly quasi-Hegelian terms as the dialect of need and demand that produces desire.

While Lacan (1975/1998) expressed skepticism about Hegelian sublation at other times, his dialectic of desire seems to make good use of the idea. In this case, need—in the sense of a physiological need such as hunger, thirst—must be addressed to the Other in the form of a demand because of the prolonged dependence of the infant. This demand, at first in cries, but then in words, is responded to by the maternal Other, who satisfies the demand or not. Because the satisfaction of every demand is reliant on the presence of the Other, the particularity of every demand is lost over time to the specificity of all demands for the presence of the Other. In this way, every demand becomes a demand for love (Lacan, 1966/2006). However, demand always represents a loss with respect to fully articulating need (Lacan, 1998/2017). Something of need is always excluded in demand in the same way something of the subject is excluded from the ideal ego. The something of need that is excluded from demand meets in the dialectic with the insatiable demand for love, creating in their sublation Lacan's conception of desire as that which is unsatisfiable and always related to lack, that which is left out of the signifying system in which demands can be articulated.

In the graph of desire, Lacan (1998/2017) developed the dialectic schematically, writing in the first level of the graph the first order of signification that represents (in part) "the mother's response" to the demand of the subject (p. 322). This response always misses something in need and leaves it unaddressed. The second level of the graph is the second order of signification that represents (in part) the "paternal presence," which Lacan described as "another instance" that is "felt beyond the mother" (p. 322). Lacan was careful to articulate that this is not about actual parents *per se*, but about the structural elements of ego formation, which his use of *instance* signals.[4] The paternal presence introduces "the mother's beyond" (p. 184), by taking the mother from the child, which induces in the subject the question of desire: "What do you want?" (Lacan, 1966/2006, p. 690).

Because of the impact of the paternal presence on the maternal discourse—how the maternal Other articulates the presence of the paternal Other—Lacan emphasized the *Name of the Father* as crucial, the Name of the Father being that which the maternal Other names as what can respond to its desire. The Name of the Father, because it separates the child and maternal Other, is the source of interdiction and prohibition—the incest taboo is established by the Name of the Father. Because the Name comes to stand in place of the desire of the maternal Other, and because it prohibits the complete enjoyment of the maternal Other, the Name of the Father—*le Nom du Père*—comes to serve also as the No of the Father: *le Non du Père*. Miller and Vanheule (2023) for this reason identify the Name of the Father as "key to the [Durkheimian] functions of integration and regulation at the heart of the social link" (p. 19). The Name of the Father, as integral to the Oedipus complex, precipitates the formation of the ego ideal at the dissolution of the complex (Lacan, 1998/2017). The ego ideal is, in this way, "what the subject identifies with when [it] goes in the direction of the symbolic" (p. 210). This is how the Name of the Father governs both integration, through identification with the ego ideal, and regulation, through the prohibition it establishes.

For Lacan, then, the ideal ego reflects the narcissistic and infantile perfection of the child based on the "relic of demand" (p. 345), that which the subject perceives the maternal Other demanding, while the ego ideal is the symbolic identification that prevents immersion in the specular image and, through the introduction of the Law, governs the subject's entry into a broader society—the family instead of a (supposed) dyad.

Bringing this Lacanian understanding of the ego ideal back to Freud, Lacan (1998/2017) built a significant amount of conceptual structure on the foundation of Freud's (1921) *einziger Zug* as an insignia of the Other, a mark delivered to the subject by the Other. It is this trait that "produces the ego ideal" (p. 286). Later, Lacan (1962) developed the singular trait of Freud into the *unary trait*, a special trait that is highly consonant with the phallus of his earlier writing (Lacan, 1998/2017) and the *Vorstellungsrepräsentanz* of Freud (1915) and which serves as a mark of an absence. It is a signifier all alone, but which initiates the child into the symbolic (Lacan, 1991/2007). Notably, the unary trait is "the commemoration of an irruption of *jouissance*," *jouissance* for Lacan being the mix of conscious unpleasure/pain with unconscious enjoyment at which symptoms are aimed (p. 77). This *jouissance* has to do with the *jouissance* irrupting into the subject prior to the imposition of the paternal Other, which is ultimately a time about which all that exists is fantasy. I will return to this fantasy later in this chapter.

For now, the connecting point between the instantiation of the ego ideal in the child, its usurpation by the leader of the group in Freud's (1921) model, and the link the unary trait serves in society is the establishment of the subject in relation to the very language that excludes it, unable to fully represent it. Just as zero is a concept subsuming no object but representing nothing within a matrix, so the unary trait marks the subject within the matrix of signification in a way that represents precisely what of the subject does not exist within the matrix, that is, what makes it unique, and this representation in language sutures the absence (Miller, 1966/1977). In this sense, the function of the proper name is also deeply connected both to the ego ideal and the unary trait Lacan emphasized later in his career. As he noted, the proper name marks something not that is a unique constellation of particularities but that:

> is irreplaceable, namely that it [what is marked] can be lacking, that it suggests at the level of lack, the level of the hole, and that it is not *qua* individual [particularities] that I am called Jacques Lacan, but qua something which may be lacking, which means that this name will be for what? To cover over another lack.
>
> (Lacan, 1965, p. 59)

Indeed, as Fink (1995) noted, "long before a child is born, a place is prepared for it in its parents' linguistic universe" (p. 5). By the time of birth, the subject is already marked by a proper name and the innumerable constructions around it that establish the relationship between this irreplaceable name and the world of signifying chains. The unary trait marks an absence, a way in which the subject is not interchangeable with other family members.

Miller (1966/1977), in his famous address delivered when he was only 21 years of age, defined the unary trait as identical to the signifier of lack in the Other. This lack, that which cannot be represented in language, is the absence of the subject, and the unary trait is a unique marking of the subject. It is the predecessor of the ego ideal, as it already introduces a disjunction between the subject and the Other, the suture of which will become the seat of a supposed unity of the name and the image (Guerra & de Andrade, 2019), and which will come to form the basis of the entrance in the social link, giving the subject an identification with respect to the Other of society.

In short, the subject assumes a unary trait that serves the function of a proper name (in Lacan's [1965] sense), a mark of what cannot be represented within language, and it is this unary trait that serves as a crucial identification for the individual and lays the groundwork for identification with the ego ideal, entering the subject into the social link. Indeed, the boundary between the unary trait and ego ideal appears thin, thanks in part to Lacan's close association of the insignia of the Other with the *einziger Zug* and, consequently, to the ego ideal. Nevertheless, the ego ideal as formulated by Freud and Lacan in his earlier period, contains a different emphasis from the unary trait as a form of name. The ego ideal is an identification with the paternal Other, while the unary trait is something that marks the singularity of the subject. To the degree that the ego ideal is a shared trait (that is, both the subject and the object of identification share it), it is not the unary trait. What permits the relation of the subject to the social link is the ego ideal, which—by suturing the subject in the signifying chain—allows the subject a method of binding libido and *jouissance* within the social link through regulation.

Even so, the unary trait's relationship to the proper name is what mediates its relevance to initiation rites. Initiation rites often involves a renaming (Van Gennep, 1909/2019), such as the taking of a Christian name in confirmation. This convention of names connecting directly to social and linguistic networks of meaning dates back thousands of years, including the ancient Egyptians (Leprohon, 2013), civilizations in the Ancient Near East, and biblical traditions of naming, such as the change of status in the signifying chain represented by *Israel* or *Abraham* over Jacob and Abram. Even though the tradition of naming has weakened somewhat in the US, names may still be a vector of unary trait identification, such as through familial name affixes, like *bat, ibn, von*, and so on. Alternatively, a given name may be important for being passed down traditionally within a family or a surname for its significance to a familial occupation (e.g., Schumacher), at least historically. In yet another form of importance, the name is also fraught for many people, such as may be the case for the surviving descendants of the North Atlantic slave trade, whose names have been lost and who at times carry the surnames of the white enslavers of their ancestors. In such cases, some may respond as did Malcolm X, who took the name X as a marker of what was missing within the language available to him (X & Haley, 1964). Similar problematics arise for those immigrants (or their descendants) who face choices about altering their names to assimilate more closely to a host culture. For example, people from cultures where the family name traditionally comes before the given name may choose to alter their name by placing their given name first in the US, and some immigrants (and others) may choose to take an "English" name to ease interactions with international audiences (Baresova & Pikhart, 2020).

Some initiation rites do not provide new names, yet other aspects provide a similar unary trait. For example, ceremonial body modification (tooth removal, circumcision) may mark one's social position within a clan or tribe, providing an ego ideal all the same (for example, by providing a view of oneself from the position of the Other of the elders). In more contemporary hazing rituals, this could be through body modification as well, but might also include garb that will mark the novitiate as being subject to a specific fraternity or sorority, and of course the Greek letters delivered to them upon accession to the group may serve as unary traits as well. Whether in the proper name, or a cough, or another form, the unary trait serves as a marker of sociality and an induction to symbolic identification.

The way in which Lacan discusses the unary trait suggests its appearance far before adolescence or the period of puberty around which initiation rites take place. The adolescent is not without a unary trait up to that point. Nonetheless, the period of adolescence is still critical in psychoanalysis as the second part of the diphasic character of human sexual life (Freud, 1905). The biological shifts of puberty bring a change in *Triebanteile*, or psychical (not biological) drive elements that are attached to repressed material (Freud, 1939). The physiological upsurge of *jouissance* in puberty marks an important instance of what Freud (1920; 1923; 1939) identified as the single connecting point of the psyche to anatomy in his metapsychology, the only violation of Freud's (1896; 1898) *as if* theoretical "speculative super-structure" (Freud, 1925b, p. 32). That is, Freud identified perception as the connecting point of psyche and physiological body, and the interoceptive experience of *jouissance* in the body is what recurs with greater strength in puberty. This *jouissance* reinforces the drive elements, pushing closer to consciousness the contents of the repressed. Freud (1905) is clear that these contents, repressed in latency, pertain to the object choice of infantile sexual life, that is, to the relationship with the Other in every sense. The unary trait, which is established at the dissolution of the Oedipus complex and establishes the incest taboo, is called into question once again in the second phase of human sexual life.[5] The social recapitulation of the Oedipal situation in initiation rites provides the enlivening of the unary trait and the incest taboo necessitated by the physiological shift. Nonetheless, the absence of initiation rites would not lead, strictly speaking, to incest. The libidinal investment in the original object has still undergone a repression in latency provided the Oedipus process occurred. Instead, the uninitiated child experiences the anxiety and *jouissance* of incestual urges and ideas in a somewhat disguised form, often appearing as a recurrence of the typical neurosis of childhood, phobia.

Taboo

Having dispensed, then, with the *totem* portion of things, this leaves the *taboo*: the prohibition of incest and the induction of the novice into the knowledge of sex. This induction typically includes two important aspects: first, it *separates* the sexes, dividing the anatomically male and female members of society, thus opening a question about the sexual difference. Second, it provides an *interpretation* of the sexual difference, usually in the form of an *illusion*. Freud (1927) defined illusions as beliefs "derived from human wishes" (p. 31), beliefs shaped by desire (although not by necessity false for that reason). Freud (1927) suggested that perhaps, "in our civilization the relations between the sexes are disturbed by an erotic illusion or a number of such illusions" (p. 34). If illusions are shaped by desire, what riper field for illusory pursuits is there than that of sexuality? In initiation rites, the novice is instructed in some way regarding marriage or the establishment of a relationship with a partner or partners predicated on the illusions of the society in question with respect to the sexual relation. The regulation of permissible object choice by society renders this induction into sexual knowledge concomitant with the incest taboo. Lacan (1975/ 1998) advanced Freud's offhanded remark about erotic illusions by formulating the notion that "there is no such thing as a sexual relationship" (p. 12), although the French *rapport* (rather than "relationship") captures a somewhat broader notion. That there is no rapport suggests not only an absence of sexual relations, but an absence of reason or of direct proportion (i.e., there is no *ratio* between the sexes; Fink, 1991).

One may, of course, protest that there is clearly a sexual relationship and that there can hardly be better evidence of this than adolescents in the throes of puberty. What Lacanian psychoanalysis attests to in stating there is no sexual relationship is that the notion of sexual complementarity—exemplified in the complementarianism of the Evangelical Christian world—is fundamentally false. There is no "opposite" sex nor Zeusian "other half," and the sexes are fundamentally asymmetrical. This is also the source of Lacan's frequent and trenchant criticism of genitality in psychoanalysis, where the notion of a mature synthesis of sexual and affective trends in the drive are united in a reproductive union of the man and the woman. How can the absence of a rapport be, given the biological circumstances surrounding sexed reproduction?

The bare nature of sex admits of a certain complementarity between the sperm and the ovum, although even this does not provide firm foundation for inductive reasoning to determine whatever could be characterized as "maleness" or "femaleness" as the characteristic of providing one end or the other of the gametic couple (cf., e.g., Koene, 2017). In humans, the picture of sexuality becomes even more complex than in animals. Where, in animals, copulation appears to be a relatively brute experience—a sort of pure phallic *jouissance* in the act, although even this is only a human construction—in humans, sex is governed by social structures. The recent social reckoning with ideas of consent reveals the power dynamics inherent in sex acts in humans that simply have no place in animal behavior. Humans place sexual behaviors in a much larger social network of exchanges and powers than anything to which animals have recourse.

Similarly, Lacan (1973/1978) observed the way in which mortality is intimately bound up with sexuality and sexed reproduction, in contrast to asexual reproduction which is an immortality of continuous self-replication. The inability indefinitely to continue one's personal existence in this life not only played a role in the development of religious rituals and beliefs but also in the secular traditions of power. The adherence across cultures and eras to laws of inheritance, most prominently in agnatic-cognatic succession, exemplifies the way in which sex is also connected to the symbolic continuation of one's existence through progeny. The importance of pedigree in the selection of sexual partners one had access to for much of history, prior to the advent of love marriage, is also an example of this. Even in the most saccharine of romances, there is typically still some residue of the social implication of the sexual relationship—the high-powered businesswoman falls for the down-home man when she's home for the holidays, or the young girl falls in love with the vampire who is afraid of exercising his power over her, and so on.

Personal power exercised in sex acts and the incorporation of sex and mate selection in social rituals of power and inheritance reflect two sides of the same issue of power in relation to sex. Beyond the social politics of power, sex is separated in myriad other ways from the supposedly evolutionarily adaptive reproductive process. In other words, the dislocation of sex from procreation has a lengthy history in human development, stretching as far back as one cares to imagine at least in the form of masturbatory behavior (Laquer, 2003). In some instances, the dislocation is directly related to matters of social structure, such as the infamous Onan (Gen. 38:1–11), who is most frequently associated with masturbation, although his sin was, in fact, *coitus interruptus*. What is often forgotten about his story is that he pulled out not because of any simple objection to impregnation (although this in itself is a layer of social reasoning above a brute instinct), but precisely because he wanted children and knew if he bore them by Tamar, *they would not be his own but his dead brother's*. The Law, not the physiological reality of insemination, would determine paternity.

Because human sexuality is so thoroughly governed by non-reproductive *jouissance* and the symbolic and imaginary structures that create it (e.g., fetishism) rather than reproduction, it is by and large "perverse," in Freud's sense, referring to sexuality with a non-reproductive end. Freud (1905) observed this facet of human sexuality quite early, writing in his *Three Essays*:

> No healthy person, it appears, can fail to make some addition that might be called perverse to the normal [reproductive] sexual aim; and the universality of this finding is in itself enough to show how inappropriate it is to use the word perversion as a term of reproach.
>
> (p. 160)

Returning to the notion of sense perception as the connecting point of psyche and soma, this connection places sexuality at the core of the mind-body nexus. Indeed, it is one's psychical response to the somatic sexual difference (both in one's experience of one's own sexuality and in the perception of the sexual difference in oneself compared to others) that is constitutional of one's clinical structure in the Lacanian sense (Ragland, 2004), that is, whether one is neurotic, psychotic, or perversely structured. Because one's psychical response may vary so widely, one's physiological experience (in the body) and psychical experience (in the mind) are not dependent on one another. This is central to understanding the distinction between the penis as an actual somatic organ and the phallus as an imaginary and symbolic aspect of psychical functioning. Ellie Ragland (2004) draws out this distinction, considering it latent in Freud's work and more fully developed by Lacan in the course of his oeuvre. The collapse of the phallus into the penis, or of psychical reality into historicism, is the error that led astray much of post-Freudian analysis, "reduc[ing] psychoanalysis to the positivistic study we now call psychology" (p. 7). Similar collapses are often found in groups that believe the creation account in Genesis is literal, that psychopathology is equivalent to neurological malfunction, or that skills-based training (that is, supposed adaptation to reality) is the highest form of psychotherapy.

Another version of this collapse, and one perhaps more easily accessible to those outside of psychoanalysis, is the collapse of anatomical sex and gender. The essentialist position asserts a tautology between the two—that sex necessarily entails gender. The real of the physiological organism (e.g., that one has a clitoris) is, in this view, a reality to which the subject must adapt. This illusory perspective is predicted on the wish for a true sexual relationship, a rapport between the sexes that is complementary, one where the body and mind are in sync and, therefore, the bodies of two sexed beings are perfectly in proportion, one seamless whole. The separation of gender from sex is a relatively new intervention at the level of social discourse (Horley & Clarke, 2016). According to this latter view, gender is a social construct that is superposed onto "the anatomical distinction between the sexes" (Freud, 1925a, p. 248).

All of this is to elucidate that the statement that there is no such thing as a sexual relationship is a condensed affirmation that human sexuality 1) is suffused with and inseparable from social constructions (i.e., non-reproductive "perversion"), especially about power; and 2) is predicated on *jouissance* rather than on procreation.

The sexual knowledge mediated by the initiation rite is its culture's illusion of the sexual relationship, which generally covers over the lack of the sexual rapport. Historically, this illusion typically contains some degree of complementarity, implicit in the separation of sexes during the process of initiation and in the different laws governing the comportment of those designated men and those designated women. The particular initiation rites of a given group also generally highlight the acceptable sexual partners one may obtain, whether one from the same religious community or specifically one from outside the totem clan in exogamy.

This leads back to the incest taboo, which encompasses not only exogamous social practices and prohibitions within the family but also the structural possibility of plenary *jouissance* in childhood. That is, the taboo is the moment of castration which forbids the subject from deriving an unlimited enjoyment from the object; only the Other has access to such enjoyment (or so the subject supposes). In reality, this experience of the incest taboo is a fundamental part of the structure of language. Because the infant is born prematurely (Lacan, 1966/2006), before it can account for its own survival, it is forced to communicate through increasingly complex linguistic formulations. The interplay of the presence-absence of the mother leads to the introduction of symbolism, wherein the word (first as crying, then later as "mama" or "dada" or the like) comes to represent the object *as absent*. If it were always present, there would be no need to have a word for it. Crucially, this language is not some natural production of an organic language acquisition device (therefore, it is at odds with Chomsky and generative grammar), but is taught by the way in which the caregivers interpret and support the behaviors, especially vocal behaviors, of the infant. It is the caregiver, for example, who decides what the significance of an infant's crying is and in what way they will respond to it. It is similarly the caregiver who typically coaches the infant in obtaining its first words. For this reason, language always intervenes in whatever paradisiacal notion of simple reality there might be; language is the intervening variable (through rules, social structures, the chain of signifiers) that precludes the possibility of there ever being a complementary sexual relationship.

Lacan identified the interdiction of the incest taboo with the *paternal function* or *Name of the Father*. This is because the interplay of the mother's presence-absence is mediated by something else she desires outside of the child, at some point discovered in the Oedipus complex as (in psychoanalytic tradition) the father. For Lacanian psychoanalysis, however, this need not be the actual father or a secondary caregiver; rather, the father's name is the crucial aspect of the function as something that is able to metaphorize—or stand in for—the mother's desire in the child's perspective. In other words, the Name of the Father is the same as the *No* of the Father (with which it is homonymous in French), such that the Name of the Father's ability to stand in for the mother's desire—that which takes the mother away from the child—is inherently also a *No*, the foundation of the incest taboo.

Because the child must pass through language in order to articulate a request for its needs to be met, and because language is always the Other's, there will always be a remainder of need that is uncommunicated and therefore not responded to in the child's address to the Other (Lacan, 1998/ 2017). Simultaneously, the presence of the Other is taken as a proof of love, such that all requests the child might make become somewhat interchangeable as what becomes sought is the Other's love (e.g., the way a child might continually want one more thing before bedtime). The Other cannot be fully and permanently present to the child, and the child's persistent request for love from the Other and the remainder of the physiological needs uncommunicated in language join together to create what Lacan (1966/2006) called *desire*. This desire is perpetually unable to be satisfied specifically because it rests on the impossibility of communication and the impossibility of a perfect love from the Other, and Freud (1931) was clear in this as well. The incest taboo is therefore a structural necessity, and the neurotic fantasy that a time before the Name of the Father exists is simply the subject's way of connecting the always already lost object of desire to its chain of signifiers.

The rite of initiation, as a sign of submission to the father's will—or in Lacanian terms, to the Name of the Father—is enacted through a symbolic castration as a mark of the incest taboo. The ritual, by psychically binding the impossibility of sexual satisfaction to a subset of forbidden sexual experiences, constructs the illusion that true sexual enjoyment is hidden behind the prohibition and may actually be obtained by some people. One example of this phenomenon is the strict sexual ethic found in certain religious groups, such as Evangelical Christians, who forbid sex before marriage; when marriage arrives, it has already been constructed as the fantasmatic point at which "at last, self-discipline is no longer needed" (Wehr, 2011, p. 93). The notion that plenary enjoyment is available beyond the limits of social laws is also revealed in the pornographic interests of the general populous, which is so often predicated on boundary violations (e.g., teachers and students, parents and babysitters, MILFs, DILFs, stepsiblings, and so on [cf. Pornhub, 2021]).

Current Trends

Psychoanalytic exploration of initiation rites surrounding puberty have lain largely fallow since the days of Reik (1915/1946) and Róheim (1922; 1942). One remarkable exception is the 2018 article by Viola and Vorcaro that takes up initiation rites in adolescence from a Freudian-Lacanian lens. They consider the transmission of knowledge of the impossibility of sexual rapport as the logical moment of adolescence. Similar to Van Gennep's distinction between puberty and adolescence, they assign to puberty all those physiological alterations in question while defining adolescence as that which "concerns the way in which the subject will address the Other and reposition himself in the social bond" (p. 2). This is because the physiological evolution of the real organism alters one's position within the social link, as do many forms of physiological or physical changes.

One of the most intriguing arguments Viola and Vorcaro (2018) make is that the crisis period of adolescence—its tumultuous rebellions, transgressions of norms, and promiscuous and perverse sexuality—is not a universal human phenomenon (unlike puberty). They attribute it, rather, to Modernity, and generally delimit it to Western societies, suggesting the concept of adolescence originated in the same cultural milieu as psychoanalysis. In their view, pubertal individuals in "traditional" societies (i.e., societies not significantly influenced by Modernism and its successors) do not experience a gap in time between childhood and adulthood. This might be illustrated by the traditional age of the bar and bat mitzvah at 12 or 13 years of age, at which point the individual is fully inducted into the community; Catholic confirmation occurring around a similar age is also notable. This might be contrasted with the American Psychiatric Association's statement on "transitional aged youth," wherein they identify "the transition from adolescence to adulthood" as the period between age 16 and age 25, a rather generous apportionment (Soe et al., 2019, p. 1). Without the gap between childhood and adulthood, the liminal rite for the novitiate is brief.

In addition to the gap of adolescence opening in Western societies, the further changes that hypermodernity has introduced into this cultural adolescent-phenomenon problematize "the family, ideals, the transmission of knowledge, and, especially, sexuality" (Viola & Volcaro, 2018, p. 2). This problematization of foundational societal elements leads to difficulties in becoming an adult—not in the physiological sense of maturation, but in the social adoption of adulthood that one can find millennials constructing as "adulting" (Madison, 2022, para 1). One might draw a comparison between the liminality of adolescence and the Lacanian tenet of prematurity at birth. From a Lacanian perspective, language, desire, drive, and ultimately culture all originate from a gross discrepancy between the physiological needs of the infant and the infant's ability to meet its own needs. Similarly, in Kehl's (2004) view, adolescence is due, among other discrepancies, to the disjunction between sexual maturity and readiness for marriage. Of course, readiness for marriage is a socially constructed matter in contrast to the physiological inability of an infant to meet its own needs; hence the universality of language in human forms of life, whereas adolescence is a culture-bound phenomenon. However, there is more to the anguish of adolescence than only this discrepancy between physiology and the social world.

One could imagine a lengthy liminal rite between the biological accomplishment of the fifth Tanner stage and the social maturity required for marriage, but one buttressed by the traditions and rituals of a given culture, ensuring the progression from child to adult in a relatively sure manner. A crucial function of such traditions and rituals, according to Viola and Vorcaro (2018), is the turning over of the body to the social link; the symbolic castration and marking of the body in these rites is critical to the socialization of the body. This social possession of the body provides limits, demarcations, and prohibitions, all binding the *jouissance* of the body. Without this binding, the adolescent's body is left untethered to the social bond and with *jouissance* unbound by sublimatory links, consistent with Freud's theories. Viola and Vorcaro put forth this untethering as causative of the adolescent's various acts upon the body (including tattoos, piercings, and non-suicidal self-injury), a matter to which Moncayo (2008) also attests. A prolonged liminal rite with sublimatory binding of *jouissance* may permit a period of non-anguished adolescence, but the disappearance of such sublimatory processes in U.S. society has rendered such a notion more hypothetical than actual for the youth of the US.

The increasing transformation of the paternal function is at play in the fading of initiation rites. In some accounts, the paternal function itself fades, leading to what some Lacanians call "new symptoms" (see Svolos, 2011) or new subjectivities (see Waitz, 2019). Without a paternal function to adequately install the incest taboo and or to provide the unary trait, the social bond begins to deteriorate. Guerra (2020) also recognized this, noting that although the Name of the Father is not excluded at the level of Oedipal processes for youth today, it is the case that the Name of the Father no longer serves as a semblant or reference point in culture. The loss of naming as a significant symbolic organization in society coincides with the loss of the naming function of the Name of the Father. Of course, the further development of Lacan of the Name of the Father into the Father of the Name bears relevance on how the loss of nomination affects the social link.

The maw of anguished adolescence has opened wide in U.S. society. The youth mental health crisis, already brewing before the COVID-19 pandemic and recently burgeoning into a nationally recognized phenomenon (Office of the Surgeon General, 2021), is a direct and observable outcome of the deterioration of the initiation rites. This has implications both for the psychical wellbeing (as loaded as this idea may be) of the adolescent as well as for society as a whole. This is because the initiation rite is intimately connected with the structure of society, as it traditionally mediates the inclusion of new members into the group.

To make sense of the clinical and social significance of the fading of these rites from U.S. society, an historical observation of the development of the current state of things is important. Only by tracing the history of initiation rites can one determine the status of youth initiation currently and chart a pathway forward that might mitigate the difficulties of youth today.

Notes

1 Freud (1921) applied this statement specifically to groups with a leader that had not achieved a degree of organization that, in McDougal's (1920) sense, would contribute to the group's accession to qualities of the individual.
2 Verhaeghe (2004/2018) commented that, in his view, "Lacan's theory is more complex [than Freud's] and takes a certain distance from the patriarchal model of Freud....The first Other is that of the body, the second Other is that of law and knowledge," and these take the place, in his writing, of the mother or father (p. 354). This erasure of sex differences is more palatable to the modern ear than to refer to the "maternal" and "paternal" Other, but it invites two problems in theory: first, it disconnects further psychoanalytic development from the bulk of human history wherein these distinctions have been meaningful, and second, it risks giving the impression—though Verhaeghe does not—that the difference in gradations of the Other is simply a matter of a supernumerary Other that is only different in sequential order without reference to the differing functions attributed to them in Lacan's theory.
3 This is a simplification, of course, as castration properly applies to the phallus. Lacan's dense, complex, and iterative development of the phallus across his three registers and the relationships between these three phalli and the *objet a*, the master signifier, and other related terms is worth its own study. However, it is not

directly pertinent here, and my own view is that the imaginary phallus is sufficiently parallel to the *objet a* in the moments of alienation and separation that I see no great harm caused by their conflation here.

4 *Instance* being the same term in French that describes the "instance of the letter" (Lacan, 1966/2006, p. 412), the "instance of the Name of the Father" (p. 483), the "three instances in the subject—(ideal) ego, reality, and superego" (p. 461), and so on.

5 While Guerra (2020) considered the intervention in this second encounter in adolescence as separate from the paternal function as established in the Name of the Father in early childhood, I treat the second intervention here as a reinforcement of the paternal function. Guerra is correct in her formulation; my treatment of it as a simpler recapitulation here is a temporary concession to slowly advancing my argument. I will revisit Guerra's conception in Chapter 7, where I will provide a fuller account of the moment of initiation.

References

Baresova, I. & Pikhart, M. (2020). Going by an English name: The adoption and use of English names by young Taiwanese adults. *Social Sciences (Basel)*, 9(4), 60. doi:10.3390/socsci9040060.

Durkheim, É. (1979). *Suicide*. G. Simpson (Ed.). (J. A. Spaulding & G. Simpson, Trans.). Free Press. (Original work published 1897.)

Fink, B. (1991). There's no such thing as a sexual relationship: Existence and the formulas of sexuation. *Newsletter of the Freudian Field*, 5(1–2), 59–85.

Fink, B. (1995). *The Lacanian subject: Between language and jouissance*. Princeton University Press.

Freud, S. (1896). Letter 84 extracts from the Fliess papers. *The Standard Edition of the Complete Psychological Works of Sigmund Freud* (Vol. I), p. 274. Hogarth Press.

Freud, S. (1898). Letter from Freud to Fliess, March 10, 1898. *The Complete Letters of Sigmund Freud to Wilhelm Fliess, 1887–1904*, pp. 301–302. Belknap Press.

Freud, S. (1905). Three essays on the theory of sexuality. *The Standard Edition of the Complete Psychological Works of Sigmund Freud* (Vol. VII), pp. 123–246. Hogarth Press.

Freud, S. (1914). On narcissism: An introduction. *The Standard Edition of the Complete Psychological Works of Sigmund Freud* (Vol. XIV), pp. 67–102. Hogarth Press.

Freud, S. (1915). The Unconscious. *The Standard Edition of the Complete Psychological Works of Sigmund Freud* (Vol. XIV), pp. 159–215. Hogarth Press.

Freud, S. (1920). Beyond the pleasure principle. *The Standard Edition of the Complete Psychological Works of Sigmund Freud* (Vol. XVIII), pp. 1–64. Hogarth Press.

Freud, S. (1921). Group psychology and the analysis of the ego. *The Standard Edition of the Complete Psychological Works of Sigmund Freud* (Vol. XVIII), pp. 65–144. Hogarth Press.

Freud, S. (1923). The ego and the id. *The Standard Edition of the Complete Psychological Works of Sigmund Freud* (Vol. XIX), pp. 1–66. Hogarth Press.

Freud, S. (1925a). Some psychical consequences of the anatomical distinction between the sexes. *The Standard Edition of the Complete Psychological Works of Sigmund Freud* (Vol. XIX), pp. 241–258. Hogarth Press.

Freud, S. (1925b). An autobiographical study. *The Standard Edition of the Complete Psychological Works of Sigmund Freud* (Vol. XX), pp. 1–74. Hogarth Press.

Freud, S. (1927). The future of an illusion. *The Standard Edition of the Complete Psychological Works of Sigmund Freud* (Vol. XXI), pp. 1–56. Hogarth Press.

Freud, S. (1930). Civilization and its discontents. *The Standard Edition of the Complete Psychological Works of Sigmund Freud* (Vol. XXI), pp. 57–146. Hogarth Press.

Freud, S. (1931). Female sexuality. *The Standard Edition of the Complete Psychological Works of Sigmund Freud* (Vol. XXI), pp. 221–244. Hogarth Press.

Freud, S. (1933). New introductory lectures on psycho-analysis. *The Standard Edition of the Complete Psychological Works of Sigmund Freud* (Vol. XXII), pp. 1–182. Hogarth Press.

Freud, S. (1939). Moses and monotheism: Three essays. *The Standard Edition of the Complete Psychological Works of Sigmund Freud* (Vol. XXIII), pp. 1–138. Hogarth Press.

Guerra, A. M. C. (2020). La nominación en la adolescencia. *Affectio Societatis (Medellín)*, 17(33), 112–132. doi:10.17533/udea.affs.v17n33a05.

Guerra, A. M. C. & de Andrade, H. V. (2019). Sobre a teoria da nominação em J. Lacan: do ato à invenção. *Tempo psicanalítico*, 51(2), 103.

Horley, J. & Clarke, J. (2016). *Experience, meaning, and identity in sexuality*. Palgrave Macmillan.

Koene, J. M. (2017). Sex determination and gender expression: Reproductive investment in snails. *Molecular Reproduction and Development*, 84(2), 132–143. doi:10.1002/mrd.22662.

Lacan, J. (1938). *Family complexes in the formation of the individual*. (C. Gallagher, Trans.). Unpublished.

Lacan, J. (1962). *Identification*. (C. Gallagher, Trans.). Unpublished. www.valas.fr/IMG/pdf/THE-SEMINAR-OF-JACQUES-LACAN-IX_identification.pdf.

Lacan, J. (1965). *Crucial problems for psychoanalysis*. (C. Gallagher, Trans.). Unpublished. https://esource.dbs.ie/server/api/core/bitstreams/2bd46730-2b17-4235-b2c6-6c5201baf6dd/content.

Lacan, J. (1978). *The four fundamental concepts of psychoanalysis*. J. A. Miller (Ed.). (A. Sheridan, Trans.). W.W. Norton & Co. (Original work published 1973.)

Lacan, J. (1991). *Freud's papers on technique*. J. A. Miller (Ed.). (J. Forrester, Trans.). W.W. Norton & Company. (Original work published 1975.)

Lacan, J. (1998). *On feminine sexuality, the limits of love and knowledge*. J. A. Miller (Ed.). (B. Fink, Trans.). W.W. Norton & Co. (Original work published 1975.)

Lacan, J. (2006). *Écrits*. (B. Fink, Trans.). W.W. Norton & Co. (Original work published 1966.)

Lacan, J. (2007). *The other side of psychoanalysis*. J. A. Miller (Ed.). (R. Grigg, Trans.). W.W. Norton & Co. (Original work published 1991.)

Lacan, J. (2017). *Formations of the Unconscious*. J. A. Miller (Ed.). (R. Grigg, Trans.). Polity. (Original work published 1998.)

Lacan, J. (2018). Note on the child. (R. Grigg, Trans.). *The Lacanian Review*, 4, 13–14. (Original work published 1986.) https://lacancircle.com.au/wp-content/uploads/2018/04/Note-on-the-Child.pdf.

Laquer, T. W. (2003). *Solitary sex: A cultural history of masturbation*. Zone Books.

Leprohon, R. J. (2013). *The great name: Ancient Egyptian royal titulary* (D. M. Doxey, Ed.). Society of Biblical Literature.

Madison, C. (2022, January 10). Doing grown-up tasks in millennial slang. *The Atlantic*. www.theatlantic.com/newsletters/archive/2022/01/doing-grown-up-tasks-in-millennial-slang/621195.

McDougall, W. (1920). *The group mind: A sketch of the principles of collective psychology with some attempt to apply them to the interpretation of national life and character.* Cambridge University Press.

Miller, A. & Vanheule, S. (2023). What holds you together: 'The social link' in Durkheim, Saussure and Lacan. *Psychoanalysis and History*, 25(1), 5–29. doi:10.3366/pah.2023.0450.

Miller, J. A. (1977). Suture. (J. Rose, Trans.). *Screen*, 18(4), 24–34. (Original work published 1966.)

Moncayo, R. (2008). *Evolving Lacanian perspectives for clinical psychoanalysis: On narcissism, sexuation, and the phases of analysis in contemporary culture.* Karnac.

Pornhub. (2021). 2021 Year in Review. *Pornhub Insights.* www.pornhub.com/insights/yir-2021#top-20-countries.

Ragland, E. (2004). *The logic of sexuation: From Aristotle to Lacan.* State University of New York Press.

Reik, T. (1946). The puberty rites of savages: Some parallels between the mental life of savages and neurotics. (D. Bryan, Trans.). In *Ritual*. International Universities Press, Inc. (Original work 1915.)

Róheim, G. (1922). Ethnology and folk-psychology. *International Journal of Psychoanalysis*, 3, 189–192.

Róheim, G. (1942). Transition rites. *Psychoanalytic Quarterly*, 11, 336–374.

Roudinesco, E. (1997). *Jacques Lacan: Outline of a life, history of a system of thought.* (B. Bray, Trans.). Columbia University Press. (Original work published 1993.)

Soe, K., Babajide, A., & Gibbs, T. (2019). Position statement on transitional aged youth. *American Psychiatric Association.* www.psychiatry.org/File%20Library/About-APA/Organization-Documents-Policies/Policies/Position-Transitional-Aged-Youth.pdf.

Svolos, T. (2011). Introducing the "new symptoms". In Y. G. Baldwin, M. Kareen, & T. Svolos (Eds), *Lacan and addiction*, pp. 75–88. Routledge.

Van Gennep, A. (2019). *The rites of passage* (2nd ed.), (D. I. Kertzer, Trans.). University of Chicago Press. (Original work published 1909.)

Verhaeghe, P. (2018). *On being normal and other disorders: A manual for clinical psychodiagnostics.* (S. Jottkandt, Trans.). Routledge.

Viola, D. T. D. & Vorcaro, Â. M. R. (2018). A adolescência em perspectiva: Um exame da variabilidade da passagem à idade adulta entre diferentes sociedades. *Psicologia, Teoria e Pesquisa*, 34. doi:10.1590/0102.3772e3448.

Waitz, C. (2019). Immersion in the mother: Lacanian perspectives on borderline states. *Psychoanalytic Review*, 106(1), 29–47.

Wehr, K. (2011). Virginity, singleness and celibacy: Late fourth-century and recent evangelical visions of unmarried Christians. *Theology & Sexuality*, 17(1), 75–99.

X, M. & Haley, A. (1964). *The autobiography of Malcolm X.* Random House.

Part II
The Disease of the Infinite

4 For the Love of God Almighty

A Brief History of the Social Link and Civil Religion in the US

The incredulity of much of the psychoanalytic community toward the bold ideas Freud communicated in his more speculative works notwithstanding, archeological and scientific research are surprisingly consonant with Freud's construction of how the social link developed in the earliest human civilizations. Already, I have mentioned the recent indications of the incest taboo's presence as far back as *Homo sapiens'* coexistence with *Homo neanderthalensis* (Sikora et al., 2017), and written legal prohibitions of incest go as far back at least as the Code of Hammurabi; the antiquity beyond memory of the incest taboo coalesces well with Freud's (1913b) suppositions in *Totem and Taboo*. Indeed, when one recalls that Freud, although writing as if the myth was about one family and about one occurrence, was intentionally condensing what he considered likely to be a recurring pattern throughout human prehistory, the grandiosity of Freud's story eases a bit. Whether he believed in the factual account or not, one can appreciate his exploration of prehistoric human psychology for what it is: a grand attempt at examining the origin of society *and its structural qualities*. Freud's (1921) supposition that group psychology is as old as individual psychology in human evolution is also a reasonable notion, as the rearing of the incapable infant during its lengthy ontogeny by powerful beings with whom it must learn to communicate (see Freud, 1910) necessitates a certain metacognitive capacity within the relationship for the individual to survive outside of infancy. There is evidence of this available in the present, such as Fonagy et al.'s (2002) notion of psychic development, wherein the child only learns to construct their own mind and emotional experiences through feedback from the parenting Other.

This connects, of course, to Lacan's (1973/1978) idea that the subject is born in the field of the Other. The psyche is structured only by the intervention of the Other—not precisely a group psychology in Freud's sense, but certainly a social field out of which the subject emerges and without which it could not be constituted. In his *Four Fundamental Concepts*, Lacan identifies the unary signifier (S1) as the signifier that represents the subject for another signifier, which is the binary signifier (S2). This formulation positions S1 as that which represents the subject in the symbolic, which, as

DOI: 10.4324/9781032666334-7

a corollary, excludes from the subject that which is not represented in it in relation to the signifying chain (S2). In its simplest elaboration, this would be those signifiers that first establish a "me" and "not-me," akin to the *Fort-Da* game Freud (1920) observed. However, this "me" and "not-me," or S1 and S2, are not indices of fact but constructions of language, and they are the minimal number of signifiers required for the birth of the subject. Freud, and Lacan following him, lay as the cornerstone of psychoanalysis that, in fact, the "not-me" is much more "me" than "me" would like to admit. This split is what leads Lacan to refer to the subject as the split subject, one consisting of both an ego ("me") in which a clear, conscious identity exists, and the subject of the unconscious. Although this is different from the question of individual and group psychologies in the sense that Freud (1921) raised, for Lacanian psychoanalysis, the subject is always born out of a social field called the Other.

If the subject is born in the field of the Other, and the social is truly at the origin of the individual, there, is reason to show interest in, rather than dismissal of, Freud's rather ambitious attempts to make sense of early psychical development as it relates to society. At the center of Freud's (1939) constructions of early human society was his belief that the earliest conceptions of deities originate in the apotheosis of earthly fathers. The totemism that was in vogue at Freud's time was, in his view, the earliest form of religion, and his euhemerism certainly echoes the work of Frazer (1890; 1910), whose work influenced Freud (1913a; 1913b; 1918; 1932; 1939).

The grand euhemeristic endeavors of the late 19th and early 20th centuries were "clearly misplaced" and overly ambitious, but Dávid-Barret and Carney (2015, p. 307) believe a narrower focus on the social function of deification would produce a more meaningful, prospective theory of why the veneration or worship of ancestors, or the elevation in death of historical figures to a place of ultimate religious honor, played a crucial role in social organization. Dávid-Barret and Carney's formal model of behavioral synchrony—a group's development of "a behavioral or cognitive state that fosters a collective action" (p. 308)—suggests that the deification of an historical figure offers significant efficiency gains in facilitating collective action for groups above a certain size. Unstructured, dyadic interactions are more efficient for small groups, but the larger the collective action, the more important that there be a single person identified as holding the truth (regardless of the "objective" truth value of that truth). The deification of such a person once dead provides a stable point of reference for the group, allowing the group to consistently reference an unchanging truth. This is consistent with the Freudian-Lacanian position that the dead father is the seat of symbolic Law, serving as a reference point to coordinate group behavior. Interestingly, Dávid-Barret and Carney hypothesize the priestly classes of religion developed as a result of certain individuals being perceived as having closer relationships with the bearer of the truth (to the dead ancestor, to the god, or so on). Given Freud's (1913) hypothesis of the familial origin of social organization, it seems worth remarking that many social groups—religions among them—use kinship cues to increase altruistic behavior within the group, such as referring to a priest as "father" or soldiers as "brothers-in-arms" (Qirko, 2004, pp. 682, 692), a matter which did not escape Freud's (1921) notice.

Moreover, the prolonged ontogeny of *H. sapiens* may also suggest the need for greater transmission of knowledge in childhood, a process that ritualistic actions may have facilitated (Nielsen et al., 2020). Ritualistic actions are distinct from ritual primarily by the lack of connection to a system of symbolization, yet they retain two other aspects of ritual: repetition and abstruseness of intent (i.e., there is no clear and immediate connection between the behavior and its outcome). Ritualistic action in *H. neanderthalensis* may have served to transmit technical knowledge even when the intent or motivation of the behavior is not immediately clear. This may have been true for early *H. sapiens* as well, although ritualistic actions and rituals became crucial for social reasons, to coordinate collective behavior, as noted above. Indeed, the ability of religion "to bind together small tribal groups" of hunter-gatherers made it an excellent mechanism for expanding and maintaining the human social bond (Whitehouse et al., 2014). Over time:

> As agriculture intensified, this ancient function [of binding small tribal groups] faded and religion became a means of reproducing much larger (if more diffuse) group identities. This entailed a change also in religion's vitality—a shift from esoteric mystery cult to something more ideologically uniform, in some ways less awe-inspiring and more controlling.
>
> (Whitehouse et al., 2014, p. 134)

The transition from binding smaller groups to larger ones corresponds both to the shift from hunter-gatherer societies (focused on smaller scale, occasional cooperation) to larger farming communities (requiring greater cooperation) as well as to the shift from infrequent, dysphoric ("frightening and/or painful") rites to more frequent euphoric or neutral rites serving less to affectively bind the group than to create an homogenous identity (p. 135). Importantly, the difference between the religious community and the social link is almost indistinguishable in early history, and the important connection between these two will be explored further below.

In the context of this information, Freud's rather ambitious suppositions may miss the historical mark in some ways, but the notion that human religion originates from the veneration of historical figures (such as leading family figures) and that these figures provide the function of organizing social groups and establishing group identity is not only not outlandish, it is supported by recent scholarship. The social link as mediated by communal religious identity based on the ego ideals of venerated ancestors and eventually gods or priests can easily be traced through history.

To take one of the most ancient examples, Sumer in the third millennium BCE was a collection of agrarian city-states (Arjomand, 2019). These city-states are among the early human communities to shift toward agriculture, where religion would begin to serve the function of binding larger social groups together as the cities became more urban, hierarchical, and specialized (Crawford, 2013). Within the Mesopotamian region at the time, "each city-state was a single temple community. The god of the city-state was its proprietor....An official called *ensi* ruled the city-state as the steward and representative of its god" (Arjomand, 2019, p. 44). Consistent with the idea of religion binding communities together, the patron deities of the city-states were, nonetheless, "all united under the overlordship of the god of Nippur, Enlil (god of storm), as the paterfamilias of an extended divine clan" (p. 44). Freud's (1939) notion that religious structure follows social structure and that polytheism (for a social structure of many separate groups of siblings) eventually gives way to "a single father-god of unlimited dominion" as society expands and consolidates central authority is reflected here in the historical record (pp. 83–84).

The structured organization of the political-religious gods and their earthly *ensis* around societal realities (e.g., city-states) reflect society's development along the lines Freud (1913) imagined when he suggested totemic deities formed initial clans and groupings. The development of human social links in the context of these ritual actions transmitting knowledge, identifications with group leaders, and proximal communities is a matter of utmost import in considering the state of the social link today.

Continuing to trace the historical journey of the social link, the cultural and religious coordination of the Sumerian cities rendered a discrepancy between the ways the city-states were unified (language, religious beliefs) and their political separation into city-states. The fragmented and fractious city-state relations, along with the cultural similarities between them, laid the foundation for Sargon of Akkad's eventual ascendancy (Arjomand, 2019). Sargon fundamentally transformed the Sumerian patchwork of city-state polities through his gradual conquest of all of Sumer. Sargon did not simply unite the city-states into a single empire, which was among the earliest of such political structures in the world. Rather, he also sought to strengthen the religious legitimacy of his reign, for which purpose he led at least one (and probably more) captured *ensi* "to the gate of Enlil at Nippur as a trophy to the national god" (p. 47), reflecting Enlil's mandate for Sargon to rule. Similarly, Sargon held himself to be the object of "divine election" and claimed domain over all of the "Land," that is, the known world (Arjomand, 2019, p. 48). In this way, Sargon co-opted the Name of the Father (Enlil) for himself as the divine ruler. Simultaneously, he claimed rights over all the world, claiming all goods for himself. This "universal monarchy" in turn constituted a "universal political community" (p. 48), a body politic united under the divine rule of a single, True King (*sharru-kin*, whence Sargon). Again, this mirrors Freud's (1939) hypothesis that the political structure of ancient Egypt following the expansion of its territory north into Syria and south into Nubia required a monotheistic turn with Atenism. In these early periods of human history—indeed for most of human history—a necessary relationship intertwined religious and political structures.

Without belaboring the point, it is also of interest to note that these sorts of developments are not unique to ancient Sumer. In ancient China, the suzerainty of the Chinese Emperor fell over everything under heaven (天下), similar to Sargon's claims over all the Land (although with debated denotative meaning; Lewis & Hsieh, 2017). The Chinese Emperors were called the Son of Heaven (Ching, 1997; Chen, 2002) and claimed to carry the Mandate of Heaven (Zhao, 2009). This evidences a similar universalizing political-religious form of link at the center of social organization, providing a legitimation of ruling powers in Chinese society (and to an extent, the societies of tributary states; see Lewis & Hsieh, 2017).

In discussing the "Name of the Father" and all the avatars of Freud's Father with a capital F, one may reasonably question why the religions and social organizations of ancient peoples were male dominated, such that both emperors and their unifying deities (e.g., the chief of the gods in polytheistic religions, such as Enlil, Osiris, Zeus, and so on) turn out to be described in language as *male*. Undoubtedly, however dubious modern analysis might find his data or principles (Hoquet et al., 2020; Tang-Martínez, 2016), Bateman's (1948) principles of sexual selection—that males have greater variability of reproductive success than females, greater variability of mating partners than females, and that the gradient of reproductive success and variety of mating partners is significant for males and not females—still have evidence supporting them (Collet et al., 2014; Jones et al., 2005). However, beyond the narrow question of whether his principles are adequate for the prediction of sex selection in a variety of animal and plant species, the logic of human mating remains a structural question. If human males benefit from a greater quantity of reproductive opportunities and females benefit from parental investment (Trivers, 1972), some degree of male control of resources (as a competitive advantage in selection) would be expected.

Ultimately, the question of the origin of masculine-bias in social hierarchies is not clearly answerable. While female sex characteristics were also represented in, for example, the Venus of Hohle Fels of the Aurignacian culture, this may or may not have anything to do with social power or with human culture subsequent to the Upper Paleolithic period. The subsequent transition in the Neolithic period from hunter-gatherer societies to agricultural ones likely coincided in Europe with patrilocality (Bentley et al., 2012), but this does not resolve the matter as matrilocality likely developed in mainland southeast Asia around the same time (Bentley et al., 2021).

In considering sex roles in social organization, Freud (1939) theorized that, once the *Urvater* was murdered, a matriarchy emerged, where the power of the father was transferred in part to the women of the horde.

Subsequently, the "matriarchy was succeeded by the re-establishment of a patriarchal order" (p. 83), although Freud did not specify how or why precisely this came about. Perhaps he may have imagined this as connected to his sexist notion that women have weaker superegos (Freud, 1925), but he does not draw this connection. The interregnum of women could easily be a pragmatic construction on Freud's part, but regardless, the cause of male hegemony is not firmly answered by Freud.

Ultimately, the cause of male dominance in the historical record is less relevant here that its consequences—the way in which the *father* became invested with a symbolic power within a diverse array of discourses in human history, at its zenith in the height of monotheistic wars of religion in the Middle Ages, often fought by men to settle the question of which man best represented the male God on earth. Without being able to answer the question of the origin of sex roles in ancient human society, it does seem reasonable to consider the construction of God as masculine or phallic to follow from the apotheosis of earthly fathers. As Lacan (1986/1992) quipped, if God made man in his image, "man no doubt paid God back in kind" (p. 196).

Whatever the source of the male image as organizing society, and however problematic this is from a contemporary perspective, deified male figures have long held positions that unified societies. Nonetheless, these historical illustrations are quite distinct from the group of practices, rituals, and beliefs that late 19th-century and early 20th-century European and American anthropologists grouped together under the heading of "totemism." As early as 1910—before Freud's (1913) *Totem and Taboo*—Alexander Goldenweiser (1910) sharply criticized the elusive nature of totemism, a term that his contemporaries used to cover a broad swath of unrelated social practices across disconnected groups. At the end of his rather extensive study, he argued for a more precise definition, even if divorced from specific practices observed. He suggested that the best definition to subsume the commonalities of the phenomena in question was: "the tendency of definite social units to become associated with objects and symbols of emotional value" (p. 275). This in itself is a stretch of the term, which is part of Goldenweiser's point. However, Freud (1913b) centered his definition of totemism on what he called "the two principal ordinances of totemism," which are the rule against killing the totem (owing to the clan's descent from the totem) and the rule against endogamy.

These ordinances can be formalized in more developed psychoanalytic terms to *identification* (with the ego ideal) and *prohibition* (of *jouissance*). Freud (1913b) believed these two functions were intimately linked because of their relation to the father in Freud's constructed prehistory. The paternal function, effecting prohibition, necessitates identification as a method of leaving behind the original object choice, at least for the neurotic. The political-religious practices of early humans and ancient peoples are of interest for their relation to identification, as human social groups organize around certain symbols, personages, and deities in a manner exquisitely consistent with Freud's (1921) ego ideal. This is the valid part of Freud's ideas about totemism, and it is the center of Freud's theory of social organization. Notably, this identification at the center of societal organization also comports with the idea that group values and practices of societies govern the protective function of integration with a society in Durkheim's (1897/1979) sense. Integration/identification with the ego ideal composes one of the two strands of the social link, following Durkheim's conception.

Taking the analysis of identification as one part of the social link further, one might also consider Jean-Jacques Rousseau's (1762/2012) tracing of the social link back to the religious practices of ancient peoples, as he argued that religion plays a key role in maintaining the social link. Rousseau described ancient deities as the definitive heads of state of early civilizations. It was in the shadow of these gods that societies organized themselves and determined their others:

> From the mere fact that people used to place God at the head of every political society, it followed that there were as many gods as peoples. Two peoples alien to one another and almost always hostile, could not long acknowledge the same master. Two armies locked in battle would not be able to obey the same leader. So national divisions gave rise to polytheism, and thereafter to theological and civil intolerance, which are naturally the same.
>
> (p. 123)

This is in line with Arjomand's (2019) account of the conquest of Sargon; while the Sumerians shared an understanding of a supreme deity, their local gods and the boundaries set on their borders made it difficult for cities to expand and intercity warfare was common. When Sargon achieved his conquest, he sought to unify the cities as the divinely appointed true king; while the henotheistic practices of ancient Sumer might permit the worship of local gods, the dominance of Enlil in the religious sphere created the cognitive groundwork to conceive of the dominance of one man in the political sphere, leading to one of the first empires in history. Also significant is Rousseau's (1762/2012) view that groups with different gods will necessarily lead to conflict. This is consistent with Dávid-Barret and Carney's (2015) argument that groups can only efficiently coordinate collective behaviors in either an unstructured, dyadic process (efficient only in small groups) or through a singular bearer of true information and those closely synchronized with that true information. With different gods, different ancestors, and different priests, groups in close proximity aligned with different true information would undoubtedly come into conflict (see Freud, 1930).

Regarding Rousseau's (1762/2012) latter point about theological and civil intolerance, Rousseau viewed the religious and the civil as essentially identical, to the point that he argued the Catholic Church (among other similar religions) was "worthless" because of the way it split the allegiance of a person between two sovereigns (p. 127). For his *Social Contract*, it seems all religion is caesaropapism—except for his vision of the Christianity of the Gospel, which was not the version of Christianity espoused by his contemporaries. What marked the Gospel version of Christianity, for Rousseau, was Christ's differentiation of religion from the State. In other words, rather than compete with the State as a temporal equal—as in ancient times, when "every State…made no distinction at all between its gods and its laws" (p. 123)—Christ's Gospel paid such little heed to the State that it did not give law the force of the supernatural, instead "detach[ing] them [Christians] from it, as from all earthly things," regarding which Rousseau quipped, "I know of nothing more contrary to the social spirit" (p. 128).

Indeed, this indifference is, in Rousseau's (1762/2012) mind, what led to the Roman persecution of Christians. Although he does not mention it, it is significant that the Romans viewed Christians as "atheists," precisely because of their refusal of the imperial cult of the Roman Empire (de Ste. Croix, 1963, p. 24). Rousseau (1762/2012) went on to criticize what a society would look like, were it actually filled with what he considered Gospel-following Christians who care nothing for the earthly kingdom; without anything tying them to the temporal sphere and to social links therein, and with such strong reverence of God's will, they would have no cause to rise up or engage in violence against their own oppressors. Of course, Rousseau (1762/2012) captures quite adequately the spirit of some Christian anarchists who see this type of society as precisely what Christ had in mind and as the reason the early Christians gave him the title Son of God, usurping the title of Augustus (see Syme, 1939/2002).

Despite Rousseau's (1762/2012) suggestion that the Gospel version of Christianity does not compete with civil powers, the argument he makes seems to be the opposite of its premise—Christianity of the Gospel and civil power cannot go together. While the temporal authority of a Crusade may compete for dominance in a way that Rousseau's Gospel Christians do not, all three modes of social cohesion (Gospel Christianity, Rousseau's Christian contemporaries, and those invested with civil power) are in competition for the loyalty of the subject, regardless of whether they identify with Christ, with the Priest, or with the Prince, respectively. In Freudian terms, despite their differences, each involves an identification with an ego ideal that determines the subject's position in the social link; they are each synchronized with a different bearer of true information.

As Rousseau (1762/2012) knew, in Europe, the conflicts of religion were far from purely spiritual. The Catholic faith of the Middle Ages gave the Pope immense temporal power far beyond a merely spiritual leader like Rousseau's Christ. Rousseau rejected the notion of the Crusades as holy war, instead suggesting that the crusaders "were soldiers of the priest; they were Citizens of the Church: they were fighting for its Spiritual country, which it had made temporal, one knows not how" (p. 130). One actually does know how, as the Donation of Pepin, the first Carolingian king, in 756 CE invested the papacy with temporal territories beyond Rome (Noble, 1984). Indeed, the papacy has consistently been interested in civil powers in Europe, whether in seeking support from various imperial factions, such as the succor of Pope Leo III in Paderborn leading up to Charlemagne's coronation as Emperor, or the struggles to wrest power from their grasp, as in the investiture controversy (Blumenthal, 1988) that laid the foundation for Italy to be rent into opposing Guelph and Ghibelline factions (see Bjork, 2010).

The common thread between the religious and secular struggles for temporal power throughout the middle ages in Europe serve to illustrate the ways in which it has been true, throughout this history, that societies organized themselves around singular leaders (e.g., the Pope) or around leading ideas (e.g., the supremacy of the Emperor), such that these identifications not only promote behavioral synchrony and collective action, but also serve to organize group violence and inter-group boundaries.

The conflation of secular and religious powers endemic in the Christian faith at the time (both East and West, in different ways) reached a new height in the Act of Supremacy 1534 (26 Hen. VIII c. 1), which established the English Monarch as the Supreme Head of the Church of England. Rousseau (1762/2012) dismissed the meaningfulness of this development, noting that subjects were still loyal to two Sovereigns (God and the monarch), with the Act not truly unifying the people under one group leader. This dismissal seems somewhat surprising, as the function of the Act merely continues, in the guise of an apparently continuous monotheism, the practice of magisterial rulers throughout history claiming to be mediators of the divine; just as the *ensi* was the mediator between a god and humanity, the King of England became the mediator of God (superseding the Pope's own similar claims).

The Protestant Reformation that was undertaken in those years is of importance in considering the social structuring of the colonies in what would eventually become the United States. The religious sectarianism that drove many of the English colonists to North America continued to characterize early colonial relations, such as the New England practice of requiring those men who would vote in the colony to make professions of faith in the church (Noll, 2006). The religious conflicts of the colonies amongst themselves reflects "the narcissism of minor differences" Freud (1930, p. 114) observed—and supports his criticism of cruel intolerance within religions generally (Freud, 1921, p. 98)—yet these differences were overcome in order to organize or synchronize the collective behavior of the colonists. While Roger Williams' (1644/1848) famous argument for religious tolerance in *The Bloudy Tenent* rather presciently argued against the use of the government to persecute people for their faith or beliefs, it took the work of many decades and many people to bring the colonists—those with power, leastways—to overcome their between-group differences. How could such differences be overcome?

Freud (1921) observed that a *leading idea* might function in place of a group leader for the libidinal organization of the group and its collective action. In his words:

> We should consider whether groups with leaders may not be the more primitive and complete, whether in the others an idea, an abstraction, may not take the place of the leader (a state of things to which religious groups, with their invisible head, form a transitional stage), and whether a common tendency, a wish in which a number of people can have a share, may not in the same way serve as a substitute. This abstraction, again, might be more or less completely embodied in the figure of what we might call a secondary leader, and interesting varieties would arise from the relation between the idea and the leader.
>
> (p. 100)

Here, Dávid-Barret and Carney's (2015) theory of deification as a mode producing behavioral synchrony again is relevant. Their conception of a priestly class developing around the truth-bearing dead leader is the epitome of the secondary leader, and Freud (1921) noted that religions in particular carry a transitional structure. From this perspective, the colonies overcame differences in some of their group identities—and "each individual…has a share in numerous group minds" (Freud, 1921, p. 129)—by recourse to a larger identification, one that could unite the colonists, including in a negative identification, that is, against the impositions of the British Crown. A leading idea entered the discourse of the colonies, that master signifier *Liberty*, to which various "founding fathers," rather plainly draped in the historical language of the ego ideal, came to play secondary leader. The irony must not be missed, of which Samuel Johnson (1775, p. 89) famously took note, that those most eager to fight for liberty were slaveholders them-selves. Without any engagement with this irony, the colonies organized around the notion of liberty, which structured their behavior and discourse, such that they prioritized the tolerance of religious and social differences within certain boundaries (showing prejudice and holding oppression still to various groups). The use of George Washington as the bearer of true infor-mation—the one who can be relied upon implicitly, who cannot lie—is clear in many ways, from the self-imposed term limit that structured the end of 30 presidential administrations to the neoclassical artwork decades later in his honor, such as Horatio Grenough's Olympian *George Washington* sculpture and Brumidi's *Apotheosis of Washington*.

That Freud (1921) considered religion the first step toward the construc-tion of a group around a leading idea is critical to understanding the devel-opment of the United States. The European monarchies continued for many more years to rely on the older form of group formation, that of an actual group leader with ultimate power, with even the French Revolution produc-ing an empire to replace a kingdom. In contrast, the United States paved its

way forward in obstinately non-monarchical efforts, presidents and politicians all performing homage, in the feudal sense, to the leading ideas of the
nation. The oaths of office, of enlistment, and of allegiance all pledge to the
Constitution rather than to any monarch or individual. This sort of abstrac-
tion requires the mediation of secondary leaders, and the early leaders
themselves became deified—the pantheon of the founding fathers. These
deified individuals embodied the abstractions of the Constitution by which
Americans were meant to live, so to speak. Much like the Roman religion
served to preserve the social link across a vast, expansive empire, so too the
United States' new religion would bind the various colonies together along
the lines that Rousseau (1762/2012) described.

Robert Bellah (1967) famously extended Rousseau's (1762/2012) conception of civil religion by elaborating the ways in which the political life of the
United States was marked by civil religion. For Bellah, as for Rousseau, civil
religion is a method of maintaining the social link. Bellah (1967) recognized
the civil religion of the United States as a product of design, discussing the
founding fathers' use of civil religion as serving a separate function to
Christianity. Bellah's immediate example of what function this civil religion
served was that:

> Under the doctrine of religious liberty, an exceptionally wide sphere of
> personal piety and voluntary social action was left to the [Christian]
> churches. But the churches were neither to control the state nor be
> controlled by it. The national magistrate, whatever his private religious
> views, operates under the rubrics of the civil religion as long as he is in
> his official capacity.
>
> (p. 46)

In other words, the function of civil religion is to permit, in the operation of
the person inhabited by the State (the magistrate, the president, the senator,
and so on), a unifying tradition that transcends the particularities of personal
piety. The unifying tradition rests upon a *deity*, not Christ by name; this is
not because the founding fathers had some abhorrence for the name of
Christ, but because the concept of the deity must be empty in order to hold
together the diverse body politic.

The empty deity of American civil religion is not one all alone; this deity still
has linkages to other parts of civil religion and certainly to society, such as
oblique biblical connections and an equality given by the Creator (a belief that
has thankfully expanded over time). The result is that particular religions may
still come into conflict with the civil religion when the links of the empty deity
come into conflict with the links of whatever deity or deities are part of a given
religion; some religious conceptions of deity fall close to the American civil
religion outlined by Bellah (1967). Others may fall further afield, leaving
adherents of civil religion with the same disposition toward the pious of
contradictory faiths as the imperial Romans had toward the early Christians.

Freud (1921) characterized groups as predicated on the foundation of love for other members within the group and "cruelty and intolerance" for those outside the group (p. 98). The dissipation of the violent convulsions in the Wars of Religion across Europe was due, in Freud's mind, not to the amelioration of the human spirit but rather the degeneration of libidinal ties to religion. Bellah's (1967) interpretation of the deity—this empty deity—as serving a unifying function provided to the American populace around the time of the Revolution a new identity under which to organize, just similar enough to each individual Christian faith so as to require minimal perceptible sacrifices on the part of the subject to join the new faith. In this view, the perception among some people today that the United States is a Christian Nation (Smith et al., 2022) is actually a reversal of the nation's initial establishment of a cult of the Republic, a civil religion in contradistinction to Christianity.

In fact, the belief that the United States is a Christian Nation, or God's country, was a later invention to strengthen national, rather than religious, identity. The reluctance of more conservative segments of U.S. society to countenance the *Götterdämmerung* of the founding fathers is more understandable when considering the role of behavioral synchrony. In this view, to reject the founding fathers, for whatever reason, is to dismiss the "true information" at the core of society, threatening the civil religion, integration in the social link, and the behavioral synchrony of the nation as a whole. This is not to suggest the founding fathers should be exempt from criticism, but to explore the broader social functions the myth of the founding fathers serves within the history of the US.

Concomitant with the decline in religious fervor in the US (Pew Research Center, 2019) has been the increasing politicization of especially Evangelical churches (e.g., Alberta, 2022). The Protestant church lacks a visible Church structure and hierarchy, such as the Vatican and its apostolic succession; even the mainline churches that ostensibly have episcopal or presbyterian polity typically recognize themselves as only one branch of a much larger invisible church, rendering the church body rather amorphous. The absence of a clear church body leaves the church, especially the corporate-modeled nondenominational megachurch segment of Protestantism, without a clear body or head, except for the Leader of the Christian Nation of America; this narrative has been pursued by one political party eager to press its advantage. The central theme of this narrative is that the body of the church is actually the body of the nation, and, thus, the group leader is not the priest (or pastor), but ultimately the President. The contours of history have led to a moment when the head of this group is so fused to person rather than office that a particular man can be said by his adherents to be President despite no longer holding the office.

Bellah's (1967) conception of civil religion has been subject to a variety of criticism, both for its apparent universality and for being the civil religion only of the white and male (Little Edwards, 2021; Remillard, 2021). Bellah

(1992) himself moved away from the term "civil religion", owing in part to misunderstandings around his intent. While the virtual cottage industry around civil religion had many issues, one point regarding the whiteness and maleness of the origin of the construct should be further considered; it is true that white men constructed the civil religion of the United States, much as they wrote the Constitution. However, at least in terms of Bellah's (1967) original paper, the purpose of civil religion was not to prescribe such a civil religion but to describe the function of civil religion in maintaining the social link (and, more particularly, to critique it). From a Freudian perspective, the singularly white and masculine nature of historical civil religion in the US might serve to highlight the cruelty of one group to those outside their group. Even so, the criticism of Bellah for initially referring to *the* civil religion misses the fact that dividing the concept of "the civil religion" into "civil religions" does not eliminate problems, it simply multiplies them (although, in fact, Bellah [1992] himself would not necessarily have agreed with this statement). In the place of one primary group, a multiplicity of civil religions would each be vying for power, each with its own leaders or leading ideas.

As it happens, this multiplicity of civil religions has been realized. The elements of a divided civil religion have been present at least since the political conflicts presaging the U.S. Civil War, but mainstream politicians since that time—the ones who have won national elections—have typically agreed on certain ideals, such as Liberty. This was especially true when the antagonism of the Cold War required a certain degree of comity between U.S. political parties, however much they might disagree on some matters. The dissolution of the social link at large in U.S. society has been visible for a period of over 20 years, although in reality this is only an acceleration of the senescence that first began to show in Nixon's administration (or, perhaps, in President Franklin D. Roosevelt's unprecedented break with Washingtonian tradition of self-limited terms). The mainstream introduction of politics based on identity in the late 20th century, and especially after the end of the Cold War, is a significant part of the process of fragmentation. Identity politics, the phrase often used to refer to this concept, is rather ill-defined and is used at times in unhelpful ways. Rather than rushing to define this term—as I think it refers to multiple phenomena—some further exploration may be beneficial.

A version of identity politics guided governance throughout the United States' history. After the Civil War, this governance appeared in numerous ways, formally in racist legal structures such as the Jim Crow laws or less formally in the extralegal terror of the Ku Klux Klan. These represent one form of identity-based political agenda. However, Lukianoff and Haidt (2018) distinguished two forms of identity politics, which they called "common-humanity identity politics" and "common-enemy identity politics" (pp. 60, 62). They first note that right-wing extremist groups, particularly those that see themselves as heirs to the Nazis, establish themselves on the hatred of various groups—a clear common-enemy identity politics. In addition, they observe that some of the rhetoric on the left has become increasingly oriented toward a common-enemy identity politics. They share as an example of this an op-ed that ran in a Texas State University student-run newspaper. The op-ed was an opinion piece decrying white people, including statements such as "I hate you because you shouldn't exist" (as cited in Lukianoff & Haidt, 2018, p. 64).[1] If one is tempted to consider the statement that white people should not exist as a symbolic deployment of "White" as a stand-in for white supremacy, one should consider the title of the essay: "Your DNA is an Abomination." This is not metaphorical language. Lukianoff and Haidt were careful to state that the response to the piece was fairly decisive, including the newspaper retracting the op-ed and firing the author, yet they observe its connection to a larger intellectual environment they tie most closely to Herbert Marcuse. In particular, they discuss what they consider Marcuse's focus not so much on liberation *per se*, but on the reversal of power structures, believing necessary the withdrawal of civil rights from some groups to ensure civil rights for others. This form of identity politics is explicitly formulated on a zero-sum understanding of the organization of the universe; it assumes that some groups must be subordinated in order for others to no longer be subordinated, and, consequently, focuses on distinctions between groups in order of priority in this zero-sum context.

This stands in contrast to what Lukianoff and Haidt (2018) cast as common-humanity identity politics, of which they consider Martin Luther King, Jr. an exemplar. In his activism for legal and political change, King (1963) appealed not to a zero-sum particularism but to the common vision of the United States. This is clear in his *I Have a Dream* speech, wherein he argues that people, both black and white, possess the unalienable rights of the Declaration of Independence. This common vision worked in conjunction with, not against, the ways in which King discussed challenges in race relations. For example, in his final book, *Where Do We Go from Here: Chaos or Community?*, King (1968/2010) called white Americans and the American government to account on racism, economic exploitation of the global south, political and financial support of racist regimes, and arguing for a guaranteed income regardless of race.[2] King maintained these positions with an emphasis on community and the ability of different groups to create a world fair for all rather than a competition between groups. In this way, King's vision pairs well with Freud's (1930) vision that cultural development should result not in a society wherein racial groups and other communities enforce their will upon other groups but in one where what would prevail is "a rule of law to which all—except those who are not capable of entering a community—have contributed by a sacrifice of their instincts, and which leaves no one—again with the same exception—at the mercy of brute force" (p. 95). Of course, this libidinal maneuver requires a sacrifice of privilege. Just as the individual sacrifices the possibility of direct libidinal satisfaction in order to achieve the protections of the group, so too the group must sacrifice libidinal satisfactions in order to achieve a higher order society that is inclusive of many diverse groups.

This vision of society as comprising ever larger groups of groups formulated only by an increasingly universal renunciation of particular satisfactions in favor of a shared ego ideal is in direct contrast to the vision of society as one wherein some groups must be excluded to an unequal degree from the levers of power. Patricia Gherovici (2022) wrote that "differences between people might be constructed tangentially on genes and biological taxonomy but are mostly about projective fantasy" (p. 186). While Lukianoff and Haidt's (2018) distinction between two forms of identity politics seems facile, Gherovici's comment could suggest a more nuanced understanding: that politics predicated on the *enforcement* of differences, that is, on their fantasmatic projections, might be distinguished from a form of identity politics that celebrates common humanity *by extending it to everyone.*

The sacrifice of satisfaction entailed in the extension of common humanity to all is not simply a Freudian matter. Abraham Lincoln, in 1838 (some 18 years before Freud's birth), delivered his Lyceum address, titled *The Perpetuation of Our Political Institutions*, in which he observed the dangers of fractious relations in the US. He viewed the fate of the US and its political institutions as predicated on how its citizenry handled submission to the law. In praising the Constitution and its application in law, Lincoln exhorted:

> Let reverence for the laws, be breathed by every American mother, to the lisping babe, that prattles on her lap—let it be taught in schools, in seminaries, and in colleges; let it be written in Primers, spelling books, and in Almanacs;–let it be preached from the pulpit, proclaimed in legislative halls, and enforced in courts of justice. And, in short, let it become the *political religion* of the nation; and let the old and the young, the rich and the poor, the grave and the gay, of all sexes and tongues, and colors and conditions, sacrifice unceasingly upon its altars.
> (p. 112; emphasis original)

This sacrifice can only be the one given in submission to the law and support of its application. Remarkably, Lincoln also draws on the importance of political religion, or what Bellah has called civil religion, in protecting and cultivating civic virtue and identity. Without the initiation of youth in the Constitution and the law—through parental transmission, teaching in schools, and so on—Lincoln foresaw the destabilization of political institutions in the US.

Lincoln's address connects the issue of social organization through identity with initiation rites in considering the transmission of such social identities to youth. In a fractious society, what does it mean to be initiated? Into which group is one initiated? The collapse of national identity in the US has left decreasingly clear what vector initiation could possibly follow. There are a number of possible pathways youth might follow in seeking initiation into some form of community, which will be discussed in later chapters, but these communities do not represent a national society nor mark a consistent transmission of group identification and regulation.

This represents a societal disintegration of which Durkheim (1897/1979) warned. Without integration, the social link itself begins to fade. It should not be surprising that Durkheim, similar to Freud (1927), observed the protective power of religion—for Durkheim, when it comes to suicide, and for Freud, neurosis. For Durkheim (1897/1979), this power was not due to the religion itself; rather "religion preserves men from suicide only because and in so far as it is a society" (p. 171). Without this community, things fall apart.

Bellah's 1967 paper on civil religion was followed up less than ten years later with a book in which he observed that "today the American civil religion is an empty and broken shell," having "been betrayed by its most responsible servants and, what is worse, some of them, including the highest of all, do not even seem to understand what they have betrayed" (Bellah, 1992, p. 142). Bellah additionally blamed the US's economic and technological advancement as having "placed power in the hands of those not answerable to any democratic process; weakened our families and neighborhoods as it turned individuals into mobile, competitive achievers; undermined our morality and stripped us of tradition" (p. 143). These statements reflect a certain pessimism about the effects of the modern world on society. Indeed, he also argued that "our ties to tradition, whatever religious or ethnic group we come from, have been enormously eroded in the last century by the advance of modernization" (p. 143). The disintegration of civil religion is due not only to the political landscape shifting over the decades but also to a concomitant fading of regulatory power of society. After considering each of these in turn—the loss of integration, regulation, and the effects of modernization and technology—I will then proceed to consider the effects of these societal changes on youth mental health today.

Notes

1 Lukianoff & Haidt note that this article was retracted and that they found it available, where it was at the time of this writing, at the following location: https://whyevolutionistrue.com/2017/11/30/texas-college-newspaper-publishes-op-ed-calling-white-dna-an-abomination.
2 Weigel (2018) was sharply critical of Lukianoff and Haidt's (2018) work; one particular criticism is the way in which she did not believe they adequately couched King's unifying language in the larger struggle for justice in which he was engaged. While Lukianoff and Haidt do reference King's civil rights efforts (how could one not?), they do not explicitly acknowledge the extent of his fights for justice. I attempt to do some of this here as I do not intend for a reference to constructive identity politics to erase the inequities that such politics were developed to address.

References

Alberta, T. (2022, May 10). How politics poisoned the Evangelical church. *The Atlantic*. www.theatlantic.com/magazine/archive/2022/06/evangelical-church-pastors-political-radicalization/629631.

Arjomand, S. A. (2019). *Revolution: Structure and meaning in world history*. University of Chicago Press.

Bateman, A. J. (1948). Intra-sexual selection in Drosophila. *Heredity*, 2(Pt. 3), 349–368. doi:10.1038/hdy.1948.21.

Bellah, R. N. (1967). Civil Religion in America. *Daedalus (Cambridge, Mass.)*, 96(1), 1–21.

Bellah, R. (1992). *The broken covenant: American civil religion in a time of trial*. University of Chicago Press. (Original work published 1975.)

Bentley, R. A., Bickle, P., Fibiger, L., Nowell, G. M., Dale, C. W., Hedges, R. E. M., Hamilton, J., Wahl, J., Francken, M., Grupe, G., Lenneis, E., Teschler-Nicola, M., Arbogast, R.-M., Hofmann, D., & Whittle, A. (2012). Community differentiation and kinship among Europe's first farmers. *Proceedings of the National Academy of Sciences - PNAS*, 109(24), 9326–9330. doi:10.1073/pnas.1113710109.

Bentley, R. A., Pradier, B., Kyaw, A. A., & Pryce, T. O. (2021). Kinship and migration in prehistoric mainland Southeast Asia: An overview of isotopic evidence. *Archaeological Research in Asia*, 25, 100260. doi:10.1016/j.ara.2021.100260.

Bjork, R. E. (Ed.). (2010). *The Oxford dictionary of the middle ages*. Oxford University Press.

Blumenthal, U. R. (1988). *The investiture controversy: Church and monarchy from the ninth to twelfth century* (U. R. Blumenthal, Trans.). University of Pennsylvania Press. (Original work published 1982.)

Chen, S. (2002). Son of Heaven and Son of God: Interactions among ancient Asiatic cultures regarding sacral kingship and theophoric names. *Journal of the Royal Asiatic Society*, 12(3), 289–325. doi:10.1017/S1356186302000330.

Ching, J. (1997). Son of Heaven: Sacral kingship in ancient China. *T'oung Pao*, 83(1), 3–41. doi:10.1163/1568532972630968.

Collet, J. M., Dean, R. F., Worley, K., Richardson, D. S., & Pizzari, T. (2014). The measure and significance of Bateman's principles. *Proceedings of the Royal Society. B, Biological Sciences*, 281(1782), 20132973–20132973. doi:10.1098/rspb.2013.2973.

Crawford, H. (2013). Introduction. In H. Crawford (Ed.), *The Sumerian world*. Routledge.

Dávid-Barret, T. & Carney, J. (2015). The deification of historical figures and the emergence of priesthoods as a solution to a network coordination problem. *Religion, Brain, & Behavior*, 26(4), 307–317. doi:10.1080/2153599X.2015.1063001.

Durkheim, É. (1979). *Suicide*. G. Simpson (Ed.). (J. A. Spaulding & G. Simpson, Trans.). Free Press. (Original work published 1897.)

Fonagy, P., Gergely, G., Jurist, E., & Target, M. (2002). *Affect regulation, mentalization, and the development of the self*. Other Press.

Frazer, J.G. (1890). *The golden bough*. Macmillan.

Frazer, J. G. (1910). *Totemism and exogamy: A treatise on certain early forms of superstition and society*. Macmillan.

Freud, S. (1910). Leonardo da Vinci and a memory of his childhood. *The Standard Edition of the Complete Psychological Works of Sigmund Freud* (Vol. XI), pp. 57–138. Hogarth Press.

Freud, S. (1913a). Letter from Sigmund Freud to Ernest Jones, December 8, 1913. *The Complete Correspondence of Sigmund Freud and Ernest Jones 1908–1939* (Vol. XXVIII), pp. 247–248. Hogarth Press.

Freud, S. (1913b). Totem and taboo. *The Standard Edition of the Complete Psychological Works of Sigmund Freud* (Vol. XIII), pp. vii–162. Hogarth Press.

Freud, S. (1918). The Taboo of Virginity (Contributions to the Psychology of Love III). *The Standard Edition of the Complete Psychological Works of Sigmund Freud* (Vol. XI), pp. 191–208. Hogarth Press.

Freud, S. (1920). Beyond the pleasure principle. *The Standard Edition of the Complete Psychological Works of Sigmund Freud* (Vol. XVIII), pp. 1–64. Hogarth Press.

Freud, S. (1921). Group psychology and the analysis of the ego. *The Standard Edition of the Complete Psychological Works of Sigmund Freud* (Vol. XVIII), pp. 65–144. Hogarth Press.

Freud, S. (1925). Some psychical consequences of the anatomical distinction between the sexes. *The Standard Edition of the Complete Psychological Works of Sigmund Freud* (Vol. XIX), pp. 241–258. Hogarth Press.

Freud, S. (1930). Civilization and its discontents. *The Standard Edition of the Complete Psychological Works of Sigmund Freud* (Vol. XXI), pp. 57–146. Hogarth Press.

Freud, S. (1932). The Acquisition and Control of Fire. *The Standard Edition of the Complete Psychological Works of Sigmund Freud* (Vol. XXII), pp. 183–194. Hogarth Press.

Freud, S. (1939). Moses and monotheism: Three essays. *The Standard Edition of the Complete Psychological Works of Sigmund Freud* (Vol. XXIII), pp. 1–138. Hogarth Press.

Gherovici, P. (2022). The lost souls of the barrio: Lacanian psychoanalysis in the Ghetto. In S. George & D. Hook (Eds), *Lacan and race: Racism, identity, and psychoanalytic theory*, pp. 183–204. Routledge.

Goldenweiser, A. A. (1910). Totemism, an analytical study. *The Journal of American Folklore*, 23(88), 179–293.

Hoquet, T., Bridges, W. C., & Gowaty, P. A. (2020). Bateman's Data: Inconsistent with "Bateman's Principles." *Ecology and Evolution*, 10(19), 10325–10342. doi:10.1002/ece3.6420.

Johnson, S. (1775). *Taxation no tyranny*. T. Cadell.

Jones, A. G., Rosenqvist, G., Berglund, A., & Avise, J. C. (2005). The measurement of sexual selection using Bateman's Principles: An experimental test in the sex-role-reversed pipefish Syngnathus typhle. *Integrative and Comparative Biology*, 45(5), 874–884. doi:10.1093/icb/45.5.874.

King, M. L. K., Jr. (1963). I have a dream [Speech]. www.npr.org/2010/01/18/122701268/i-have-a-dream-speech-in-its-entirety.

King, M. L. K., Jr. (2010). *Where do we go from here: Chaos or community?* Beacon Press.

Lacan, J. (1978). *The four fundamental concepts of psychoanalysis*. J. A. Miller (Ed.). (A. Sheridan, Trans.). W.W. Norton & Co. (Original work published 1973.)

Lacan, J. (1992). *The Ethics of Psychoanalysis* (J. A. Miller, Ed., D. Porter, Trans.). W. W. Norton & Co. (Original work published 1986.)

Lewis, M. E. & Hsieh, M. Y. (2017). Tianxia and the invention of empire in east Asia. In B. Wang (Ed.), *Chinese Visions of World Order: Tianxia, Culture, and World Politics* (pp. 25–48). Duke University Press.

Lincoln, A. (1838). The perpetuation of our political institutions. *Collected Works of Abraham Lincoln* (Vol. I), pp. 108–115. Rutgers University Press.

Little Edwards, K. (2021). Seeing Bellah's Civil Religion through a Black Feminist lens. In R. H. Williams, R.HaberskiJr., & P. Goff (Eds), *Civil Religion Today: Religion and the American Nation in the Twenty-First Century*, pp. 95–117. NYU Press.

Lukianoff, G. & Haidt, J. (2018). *The coddling of the American mind: How good intentions and bad ideas are setting up a generation for failure*. Penguin.

Nielsen, M., Langley, M. C., Shipton, C., & Kapitány, R. (2020). Homo neanderthalensis and the evolutionary origins of ritual in Homo sapiens. *Philosophical Transactions of the Royal Society of London. Series B. Biological Sciences*, 375 (1805), 20190424–20190424. doi:10.1098/rstb.2019.0424.

Noble, T. F. X. (1984). *The republic of St. Peter: The birth of the Papal State, 680–825*. University of Pennsylvania Press.

Noll, M. A. (2006). British and French North America to 1765. In S. J. Brown & T. Tackett (Eds), *The Cambridge History of Christianity* (Vol. VII), pp. 392–410. Cambridge University Press.

Pew Research Center. (2019). In US, decline of Christianity continues at rapid pace. Pew Research Center. www.pewresearch.org/religion/2019/10/17/in-u-s-decline-of-christianity-continues-at-rapid-pace.

Qirko, H. (2004). Altruistic celibacy, kin-cue manipulation, and the development of religious institutions. *Zygon*, 39(3), 681–706. doi:10.1111/j.1467-9744.2004.t01-1-00608.x.

Remillard, A. (2021). Regions and Civil Religion(s) in America. In R. H. Williams, R. Haberski Jr., & P. Goff (Eds), *Civil Religion Today: Religion and the American Nation in the Twenty-First Century*, pp. 76–94. NYU Press.

Rousseau, J.-J. (2012). *Of the social contract and other political writings* (C. Bertram, Ed., Q. Hoare, Trans.). Penguin Classics. (Original work published 1762.)

Sikora, M., Seguin-Orlando, A., Sousa, V. C., Albrechtsen, A., Korneliussen, T., Ko, A., Rasmussen, S., Dupanloup, I., Nigst, P. R., Bosch, M. D., Renaud, G., Allentoft, M. E., Margaryan, A., Vasilyev, S. V., Veselovskaya, E. V., Borutskaya, S. B., Deviese, T., Comeskey, D., Higham, T., … Willerslev, E. (2017). Ancient genomes show social and reproductive behavior of early Upper Paleolithic foragers. *Science (American Association for the Advancement of Science)*, 358(6363), 659–662. doi:10.1126/science.aao1807.

Smith, G. A., Rotolo, M., & Tevington, P. (2022, October 27). Views of the U.S. as a 'Christian nation' and opinions about 'Christian nationalism'. Pew Research Center. www.pewresearch.org/religion/2022/10/27/views-of-the-u-s-as-a-christian-nation-and-opinions-about-christian-nationalism.

de Ste. Croix, G. E. M. (1963). Why were early Christians persecuted? *Past & Present*, 26, 6–38.

Syme, R. (2002). *The Roman revolution*. Oxford University Press (Original work published 1939.)

Tang-Martínez, Z. (2016). Rethinking Bateman's Principles: Challenging persistent myths of sexually reluctant females and promiscuous males. *The Journal of Sex Research*, 53(4–5), 532–559. doi:10.1080/00224499.2016.1150938.

Trivers, R. (1972). Parental investment and sexual selection. In B. G. Campbell (Ed.), *Sexual selection and the descent of man 1871–1971*, pp. 136–179. Aldine Publishing Company.

Weigel, M. (2018). The Coddling of the American Mind review – how elite US liberals have turned rightwards. *The Guardian*. www.theguardian.com/books/2018/sep/20/the-coddling-of-the-american-mind-review.

Whitehouse, H., Mazzucato, C., Hodder, I., & Atkinson, Q. D. (2014). Modes of religiosity and the evolution of social complexity at Çatalhöyük. In I. Hodder (Ed.), *Religion at Work in a Neolithic Society*, pp. 134–156. Cambridge University Press. doi:10.1017/CBO9781107239043.008.

Zhao, D. (2009). The Mandate of Heaven and performance legitimation in historical and contemporary China. *The American Behavioral Scientist (Beverly Hills)*, 53(3), 416–433. doi:10.1177/0002764209338800.

5 The Impact of Consumer Capitalism on the Social Link

Lacan was not always aligned with Freud with respect to the various formulations he had regarding the father—particularly with respect to the Oedipus complex and the *Urvater*. Lacan (1991/2007), after a certain time, suggested interpreting the Oedipus complex as Freud's "dream" (p. 117) and called *Totem and Taboo*, the work perhaps dearest to Freud (Strachey, 1955), "*Totem and Total Bull*" (Lacan, 2011/2018, p. 184) and "Darwinian buffoonery" (Lacan, 1991/2007, p. 112). Nevertheless, Lacan did not abandon the underlying ideas involved in these myths. Rather, he undertook a reduction of the myths to their structural cores. Lacan did this primarily through his formalization of analytic ideas in his algebra. This includes the $\math$, S1, S2, and a of the previous chapter, but his development of them went further.

Lacan's formalization of the structure of Freudian theory is essential to the consideration here of the effects of consumer capitalism on initiation rites and the social link in the 21st century. There has been too much written on Lacanian theory and economics already, especially from the perspective of Marxism, a discourse as bound as capitalism to the master signifier of the market (Lacan, 1991/2007). This chapter does not aim to offer an economic critique, much less to lionize some particular economic model (whether capitalism, communism, socialism, or something else). Rather, the narrow focus I take here is on the effects of consumer capitalism on the social link. However, in common with other post-Lacanian literature, Lacan's conception of discourse is a fundamental bedrock to any discussion of the social link.

"Discourse" is a word widely used in Lacanian psychoanalysis, although not always consistently. There are two primary ways in which the word seems to be employed, corresponding to Lacan's own evolving use of the term over the course of his seminar. They are:

1   Discourse as any structured set of signifiers functioning as a social link. For example, Lacan might refer to "*discours scientifique*" in this sense, and it is also found throughout his body of work.
2   Discourse as one of four designated and specific structures, comprising four terms, that Lacan (1991/2007) first introduced in *The Other Side of*

DOI: 10.4324/9781032666334-8

Psychoanalysis. In this sense, the term is one of controlled vocabulary, identifying only four canonical discourses that combine the four terms.

(Lacan, 1972, p. 23)

Lacan (1972) offered a specific definition of discourse later in his career, which seems apropos to both above usages: "*Le discours c'est quoi? C'est ce qui, dans l'ordre... dans l'ordonnance de ce qui peut se produire par l'existence du langage, fait fonction de lien social*" (p. 23). Discourse is what, in the ordering of that which can be produced by the existence of language, acts as a social link. This definition seems to incorporate both of the ways Lacan uses the term discourse, and both uses appear even in the context of the same lecture from which this definition is taken.

That discourse acts as a social link for Lacan directly connects the Durkheimian social link—comprising integration and regulation—with Freudian-Lacanian theory. Discourse is what governs in some way both an identification within the link as well as a regulation of desire. Lacan's four canonical discourses, and a fifth one he added later, are central to the investigation of the social link from a Freudian-Lacanian perspective.

Each of Lacan's four discourses comprise a constellation of four terms— the same four terms are in each discourse, although in different positions. The four terms are: S1, S2, $, and *a*, all elements of the Lacanian algebra he developed for many years as a formalization of his thinking. As noted in the previous chapter, S1 and S2 are the minimum signifiers required for the birth of the subject. However, Lacan (1991/2007) went on to elaborate S1 and S2 further. For Lacan's formulations in the four discourses, S1 becomes the master signifier, the signifier that structures and organizes the social link. This same S1 that Lacan called the unary signifier at the time of the *Four Fundamental Concepts* (Lacan, 1973/1978) he called in *The Other Side* (Lacan, 1991/2007) the unary trait—that organizing trait both of the subject's psyche as well as of the social link. This version of the unary trait is a direct heir to Freud's (1921) *einziger Zug*, a point of identification that also places one in the context of the universe of signifiers.

The S2, likewise, is somewhat expanded, primarily as an encapsulation of knowledge that "initially stems from the unary trait and, in its wake, from everything that can possibly be articulated as signifier" (Lacan, 1991/2007, p. 50). S2 is a knowledge that follows from S1 or is permitted by S1. Thus, as for the subject, so too for discourse—there must always be at least these two terms (Lacan, 1972).

The $ is the subject as split or divided between conscious and unconscious, that which is represented and that which is unrepresented. The final term, *a*, is related to the lost object-cause of desire discussed in Chapter 3; however, Lacan additionally invested this term with that which the subject experiences in losing *jouissance* through the imposition of the S1, namely, surplus *jouissance*. That is, the relationship between the unary trait (S1) and the knowledge it organizes (S2) creates a structure that situates the subject

(S) with respect to the Other's *jouissance* (a), a *jouissance* that opens up through the perception of a loss (Lacan, 1991/2007, p. 51). Lacan's deployment of surplus *jouissance*, as a concept borrowed from Marx's surplus value, reflects that the subject's labor entering into language results in a loss of *jouissance* that executes a forever loop, leading the subject always to repeat in order to refind the surplus *jouissance* lost in language. This is how Lacan read Freud's lost object as the lost object-cause of desire and what motivates, in part, the repetition.

Fundamentally, the four discourses mark differing structural arrangements of these four terms. These discourses are an undeniably structuralist intervention by Lacan, reflecting the unfolding of certain laws, or structural necessities, of language that simply cannot but be as they are (Lacan, 1991/2007). One aspect of this structural unfolding is the description of four positions through which the four terms dance.

In the first iteration of these positions, Lacan characterized them as, on the left, Desire over Truth, and on the right, Other over Loss (Lacan, 1991/2007, p. 93). This reflects that the dominant position, that of the upper left, encapsulates a certain desire, which—by virtue of the structure that leads an arrow from this position to the Other—is the representation of Lacan's dictum from his early seminars that "man's desire is the desire of the Other" (Lacan, 1991/2007, p. 93). Here, the positions underneath the bars are a position of repression, indicating that desire represses a truth and that the Other represses a loss of *jouissance*, from which surplus *jouissance* springs.

As might be gathered by the elaboration of these positions, the four discourses are not only descriptive of the social bond but reflect solutions to the question of sexual non-rapport, or sexual knowledge (Lacan, 1991/2007; Vanheule 2016). Put another way, every social bond is a method of accounting for the loss of *jouissance* that results from the imaginary genital relation—social bonds are a way to bind and manage *jouissance* within the context of a meaning. This is why the transmission of a fantasy in initiation rites governs sexual behavior, by establishing a myth that rectifies the incommensurability of humanity with nature.

These ideas become somewhat clearer as one follows Lacan's refinement of his four positions. Later, in the same year of his seminar that he outlined the initial positions, Lacan (1991/2007) elaborated the following positions: Agent over Truth to the left of Work over Production (Lacan, 1991/2007, p. 169). This organization of positions reflects perhaps his most frequently cited account of the structure of discourse, and it contains some clarifications.

Although truth is retained, desire becomes agent, reflecting not an agent of pure autonomy as one might expect in English, but with the ambiguity of an agent whose agency is caused—in this case, by that which remains the same, the truth that the agency hides (Lacan, 1991/2007, p. 199). Work, rather than the Other, appears on the top right, which reflects the agent seeking to put something to work in order to achieve a production. The relationship between Other and work has to do with the labor of the Other, that is, of the subject's entrance into language, and the loss—and creation—of *jouissance* that is the production of such labor. Thus, loss and production are also closely comingled, one causing the other.

Finally, in …*Ou Pire* two years later, Lacan (2011/2018) elaborated the following, less frequently cited positions: Semblance over Truth to the left of *Jouissance* over Surplus *Jouissance* (Lacan, 2011/2018, p. 169).

Here, truth again remains victorious in keeping its position, although once again, the terms that come into play in the other three positions are all closely related to their antecedents. The relationship of semblance to agent and to desire has to do with Lacan's evolving use of the term *semblance*. Semblance, by the time of his work on discourses, comes to hold the position of that upon which discourse is founded (Lacan, 1971; Vanheule, 2016), and in particular, the fact that the Name of the Father, once undergirding the social bond and the psyche in Lacan's thinking, comes to occupy a place in which the Father is no longer real but operates nonetheless as a guarantor of the social bond as a semblant (Grigg, n.d.). The distinction here between an ontologically heavy Name of the Father and a paper tiger Name of the Father seems to be fairly thin; whether one considers the Name of the Father as real or merely an artifice, its relationship to the social bond remains the same, without difference. This is an identical circumstance to Lacan's (1966/2006) averment that "there is no Other of the Other" (p. 688) while at the same time holding the operation of *separation* as critical in subjectivity (which necessitates the Other of the Other as that which causes the disjunction between the Other's object of *jouissance* and the subject).

Nevertheless, Lacan's placement of semblance in the position of dominance reflects the key role that the semblance plays in discourse. For Lacan (1971) all discourse is predicated on a semblance; he summarized the entirety of the 18th year of his seminar, *On a discourse that might not be a semblant*, by saying he "spent the year demonstrating that this discourse is altogether excluded" (Lacan, 1972, p. 11), that is, there is no discourse that might not be a semblance. All discourses are based on a fantasmatic ironing out of the sexual relation, although the analyst's discourse is somewhat different to the extent that it seeks not to utilize power but to proceed through a series of half-sayings toward the truth.

Returning to Lacan's (2011/2018) third account of the positions of discourse, the superposition of *jouissance* and surplus *jouissance* in the place of Other/work and loss/production, respectively, again suggests the consonance of these ideas throughout Lacan's trajectory in elaborating the terms. The *jouissance* of the Other, the work of entering language that entails a certain "*jouis-sens*" (Lacan, 1974/1990, p. 10) or enjoyment of meaning, also produces the loss that engenders the surplus *jouissance*.

What is most remarkable about Lacan's (2011/2018) revision in …*Ou Pire* is his addition of arrows across most of the terms in the discourses; for example, one can see the vectors displayed in this version of the master's discourse from ...*Ou Pire* (p. 207). These arrows show the utter incommunicability between the truth and its partner on the lower register (Lacan, 1991/2007, p. 174), as no arrow connects the place of truth to the produced loss engendering surplus *jouissance*. What relations are marked are those between the remaining positions.

The arrow from desiring agent and semblance (top left) to the Other of labor and *jouissance* (top right) remains in place, suggesting the way in which the semblance, hiding its cause (truth; bottom left), makes an effort to address the non-rapport of the sexes, which is itself brought about by the labor of *jouissance* one imagines in the Other as an historical occurrence. There are four new arrows: one extending from truth to semblance, which it causes; one extending from truth to *jouissance*, which it shapes; one extending from surplus *jouissance* produced by loss back to the semblance which animates desire and transverberates the subject; and one extending from the Other of labor and *jouissance* to the produced loss and surplus *jouissance*.

These arrows denote a stable, structural course that constitutes a circuit. What powers the circuit, one might intuit, is that which has no other connection to discourse than those leading away from it, namely, truth. The truth does not enter the fray, giving it a privileged position as a stable point from which the other positions obtain. This also means that there is a lack inherent in the circuit; the truth is never fully integrated. The circuit runs from the truth to the semblance, from both to *jouissance*, and from *jouissance* to surplus *jouissance* which leads back to the semblance. This reflects that:

1   The truth is always half-said and never full.
2   The truth is the cause of the semblant.
3   The system is stabilized in its flow because of the steady secretion of truth through the system without being incorporated thereby.

The relationship of truth as a stabilizing force in discourse is a central and overlooked aspect of Lacan's theory of discourses. That the truth is always half-said is not coincidental to the nature of truth but essential to it. This is the truth of the split subject (S) that is not-all contained within the signification that represents it in the signifying chain; it is the truth of sexual rapport, which is never fully genital or oblative, nor fully captured within the action of reproduction. That this fundamental incompleteness should serve as a brake on discourse and the social link is due to the organization of society around true information. When there is room within discourse for an incompleteness, it is less likely for there to be excesses in governance. Consider, for example, Durkheim's (1897/1979) hypothesis regarding regulation. Durkheim wrote that regulation of desire was necessary in society; in contrast to animals, whose relative lack of metacognitive ability precludes ambition in the human sense, humanity is unbounded in its ambition for better conditions. However, there is a natural limit to this ambition such that the barriers of the real preclude further development. Despite this natural limit, "nothing appears in man's organic nor in his psychological constitution which sets a limit to such tendencies" (p. 247). Nothing within the individual bounds the limits of ambition, which anticipates Freud's (1930) reflection that this sort of eternal possibility of improvement must be sacrificed on the altar of society for security. From Durkheim's (1897/1979) view, however, it is not so much for security from oppression by the powerful that one must sacrifice; it is because not having a limit imposed leads to untenable results. "Unlimited desires are insatiable by definition and insatiability is rightly considered a sign of morbidity. Being unlimited, they constantly and infinitely surpass the means at their command; they cannot be quenched. Inextinguishable thirst is constantly renewed torture" (p. 247). This philosophy of desire is strikingly consonant with Lacan's own theorization of desire as going beyond the bare satisfaction of instincts that animates animal life and is always operative as that which has no object such that it could be satiated.

The truth of insatiability is negotiable in the social link—in discourse—only by the work of the semblant, which organizes society and constructs a fantasy around lack. In this way, a society can support stabilization and regulation through an account of lack that incorporates it into the system, such as traditions around licit sexual behaviors or theological constructions inclusive of negative theology. This is how societies prevent the burnout of untamed desire.

The positions Lacan developed in his account of discourse are central to understanding consumerism, even more so than the terms that perform their dance through them. This is because the directionality of the vectors Lacan established were revised in 1972, when he contributed an additional, fifth discourse, going against his own supposition that the four discourses are the complete set of structural arrangements. He called this fifth discourse the discourse of the capitalist. In addition to altering the position of the terms (he placed them out of order, no longer merely rotating them) he also changed the vectors connecting each of the positions.

In the capitalist's discourse, which Lacan (1972) called the "substitute" of the master's discourse (p. 20), the position of S1 and $ are swapped (compared to the master's discourse). Moreover, the arrow between the semblance and *jouissance* has been erased, and the arrow connecting the semblance and truth has been reversed, such that truth is no longer the cause of the semblance. The resulting circuit has none of the characteristics enumerated above regarding the vectors. In opposition to them:

1   The truth is assumed in the system as fully said.
2   The truth is not the cause of the semblance but pulled into the discourse as created by the semblance.
3   The system is destabilized because lack is not incorporated into the system such that it allows for a brake.

Regarding this last point, Lacan stated that the discourse is "headed for a blowout" because "[it] goes on casters, indeed [it] cannot go better, but [it] goes too fast, [it] consumes itself, [it] consumes itself so [it] is consumed" (Lacan, 1972, p. 20). Because the arrows all lead one to the other, the circuit fully integrates every element and has no brakes. The capitalist discourse proceeds, then, from a dominant position of the split subject (S) seeking the S1 that could complete it—in other words, seeking a demand that could perfectly enunciate need such that no desire would persist. This S1, in the position of truth, leads to the *jouissance* of the S2, a series of knowledges meant to satisfy the demand of the subject. Alas, this only produces the surplus *jouissance* (a) resulting from loss as each S2 in the series fails to provide plenary satisfaction. This leads back to the start of the symmetrical discourse, beginning again with the demanding subject without break.

While Lacan called this the capitalist discourse, this does not necessarily coincide with a capitalist economic structure as such, in my view; private ownership of the means of production has little direct bearing on the role truth plays in discourse. Consumerism, however, relies on the structure of truth in discourse, as do other ideological constellations, and I share Stavrakakis's (2007) view that consumerism is especially part of late-stage capitalism. Taking the fifth discourse as a consumerist discourse, the position of S1 in the place of truth suggests an assumption of wholeness as the central truth of the social link; if you are not whole, it is a flaw in the system. While this position is shared with the university discourse, the circuit is altered in the fifth discourse such that this becomes the full truth; within this social link, there is no lack. The knowledge (S2) in question in this discourse is, in the consumerist case, most exemplified in the brand name or the image conveyed by brand messaging.

Consumerism itself would hit a natural limit of profitability if it were restricted to the actually possible. The introduction of technologies capable of inflaming imaginary passions, such as photo editing software and television, and most recently so-called artificial intelligence, have created the foundation of the fifth discourse as one in which desire is not permitted. The assumption of truth as fully said and as constructed by the semblant (rather than the truth causing the semblant) is immediately detrimental to regulation in the social link as the perpetual renewal of the demand (rather than desire) always moves the boundaries of the socially acceptable. While ideologies and religions have previously asserted dominance in the world through relatively stable regulatory principles, technology has given rise for the first time to a system that can simultaneously exert pressure on hundreds of millions of persons in one instant. This weakens the power of traditional analogue mediations of regulation and strengthens the power of imaginary regulation based upon the conformity of the subject to the image presented through digital media.

Without the meaning of the fantasy provided by the semblant that hides and mediates the truth, there is a distinction that deteriorates. This distinction is the one between lack as a structural law and loss as a matter of history.[1] While the fantasy in, for example, the master's discourse always provides a narrative of loss that articulates the truth of lack, such a fantasy typically involves a degree of acceptance regarding lack. For example, consider the very literal taboo upon incest; the regulation of sex behavior by the principle of the incest taboo constructs a narrative of loss (one must leave the family) in a way that incorporates lack as a definite feature (the divinity has prohibited incest, so it is not negotiable). In other words, loss and lack arrive together, with loss adorning lack and making it somewhat palatable. Although incest is prohibited, you could have a substitute satisfaction through the regulation provided by the semblant.

The four original discourses delimit sexual non-rapport through a strategy that embraces loss (of *jouissance*) because of the truth's presence as lack, as only half-said and not entered into the circuit. The loss embraced in these discourses is what Lacan developed in ...*Ou Pire* (Lacan, 2011/2018) and *Encore* (Lacan, 1975/1998), namely, that everyone has undergone the phallic function and yet there is at least one who has not undergone the phallic function. In other words, the subject within the four social links mediated by Lacan's four discourses must accept the fact that *some* sexual rapport is forbidden or withheld *by the Other*; as a consolation prize, the subject has access to aim-inhibited substitute satisfaction. This is entirely consistent with Freud's (1930) understanding of the social bond, wherein civilization can only function through such substitution. The substitutive satisfaction is available to the subject to the extent that it assumes a fantasmatic construction of sexual rapport, that is, the fundamental fantasy Lacan (e.g., 1998/2017a) documented as $S \lozenge a$, the split subject in relation to the partial object (cause of desire) that one imagines could be satisfactory. This is why Lacan can speak of surplus *jouissance*. The relationship between the *jouissance* imagined as lost and the *jouissance* of the present is like the relationship between the first high, which one chases with every subsequent use of substances, and the most recent one that never quite attains the same level of satisfaction. The drive for *jouissance* chases the imaginary first satisfaction, as if—if only the right conditions are met—the subject could experience satisfaction.

Thus, the novice is initiated into a society wherein certain *jouissance* is forbidden by the Other, but not all *jouissance*. While the compromise entails a loss of *jouissance* (although this loss occurs only in fantasy), it is also true that it binds surplus *jouissance* within the social tie such that it loses its horrifying and overwhelming character. Lack is *necessary* at the center of this process, that is, necessary in the sense Lacan (2011/2018) uses it, in reference to the idea that "there exists an x determined by having said no to the phallic function," which he notates $\exists x \overline{\Phi} \overline{x}$ (p. 178). This notation is one of four such formulae Lacan developed in the 19th and 20th years of his published seminar. The relation between the $\exists x \overline{\Phi} \overline{x}$ and the four discourses may seem obtuse at first, but to separate these two developments (the four discourses and the four formulae) in the later period of Lacan is to misread both of them.

The discourses are inseparable from the body; despite the abstract way in which some theoreticians deploy these discourses as essentially incorporeal social factors, they are still *en corps*. The foundation of the discourses is the body, which renders a much more grounded sense of what is at stake in each of the discourses acting as social links. Lacan (2011/2018) centered the emergence of the quaternary structure of the discourses—regardless of the terms passing through the four positions—in *jouissance* experienced in the body. *Jouissance* plays the role of the originating principle of the structure of discourse, arising first "as something that is ungraspable" (p. 202). In other words, the experience of *jouissance*, which is at once enjoyment and suffering, is ungraspable by the subject, such that "the other three [positions] rise up" to structure the experience (p. 202). This is the structural, Lacanian understanding of Freud's (1930) hypotheses about libido's centrality to the social bond, both as something that motivates the social bond in its aim-inhibited form, but also that which degrades and endangers the social bond when the libido is not bound in an aim-inhibited manner. Lacan, despite levying several critiques of Freud by that point of his career, is nonetheless not shy about directly connecting his account to Freud.

For Lacan (2011/2018), the first position to arise after *jouissance* is truth; "truth already implies discourse," despite that it cannot be said (p. 202). Furthermore, "for *jouissance* to exist, one has to be able to speak about it," speak about it even if the truth is unsayable; there is always "*the fact of saying*" that is entailed in the response of truth to *jouissance* (p. 202). As Lacan put it:

> The fact of saying has its effects, on the basis of which what is known as the fantasy is constituted. The fantasy is the relation between the object a—which is what is concentrated through the effect of discourse in order to cause desire—and this something that is condensed around it, as a split, and which is called the subject.
>
> (pp. 205–206)

This relates to the $\exists x \bar{\Phi} \bar{x}$ precisely because "we can say absolutely nothing that resembles anything that might constitute a truth function if we do not admit the necessity of *there being at-least-one who says no*" (Lacan, 2011/2018, p. 184). For truth, the driving force of discourse in response to *jouissance*, to exist, there must necessarily be $\exists x \bar{\Phi} \bar{x}$. Lacan is clear that this one who says no is the father, not only because his name is No (*le nom/non du père*), but because the saying no is the function of the father (p. 184). Lacan acknowledges, however, that "it's not inevitable that he should be the father in flesh and blood," and confidently stated that "there is always one" who will fill the function of the father, to "wow" the family (p. 184). It is the wowing power of "no" that constitutes lack in the subject through the function of separation (or the recognition of this wowing in the discourse of the Other). The prohibition is what allows the subject to suppose that plenary satisfaction would have been possible if only it had been permitted (which is the function of loss), despite the fact that the prohibition itself is only a product of structure, such that true satisfaction is not only unattainable but oxymoronic (which is the function of lack).

Thus, lack is necessary for the functioning of the four discourses. Discourse can only operate with the mobilizing truth when there is an operating paternal function that can bind *jouissance* through the provision of all the materials necessary for a fundamental fantasy. This is what Lacan (2011/2018) meant when he said that "discourse as such is always a discourse of semblance, and…if there is something at some point that is authorized by *jouissance*, then this is precisely the fact of affecting a semblance" (p. 202).

The fantasm that marries loss and lack—the perceived loss of *jouissance* with its structural impossibility—gives an excuse within the social bond for why total satisfaction is not permissible. This is crucial, because it socializes and binds the acceptance of loss as the price of entrance into the social link, effecting both integration and regulation in one moment. Loss is colored with the lens of necessity, and desire is an indelible part of discourse. This is why Lacan's (1998/2017a) most concise definition of the fantasy is "the imaginary captured in a particular use of signifiers" (p. 387).

However, this does not apply for the fifth discourse. Because truth is assumed to be fully said within consumerism, that is, all of need can be articulated in a demand and satisfied, structural lack is completely removed from the circuit (as truth is fully incorporated, or incorporated as full). This is why, some months before his elaboration of the formula of capitalist discourse, Lacan (2011/2017b) described that:

> What differentiates the discourse of capitalism is *Verwerfung* [foreclosure], the fact of rejecting, outside all the fields of the symbolic. This brings with it the consequence I have already said it has. What does it reject? Well, castration. Any order, any discourse that aligns itself with capitalism, sweeps to one side what we may simply call, my fine friends, matters of love.
>
> (pp. 90–91)

Consumerism thrives on the formal elimination of desire, such that the subject falls again and again for the lure of the demand. There is only loss that can and must be redressed; there is no lack inherent in the existence of the speaking being. The erasure of lack is directly connected to the fading of the paternal function, and with no paternal function, there is no ground for a truth function. There is a direct link between consumerism and "post-truth" society (which is not so different from a postmodern one). The role of the paternal function in establishing an exit from an untenable circuit is something clear as early as *Formations of the Unconscious*, wherein Lacan (1998/

2017a) elaborated his graph of desire in such a way that the second stage, which he called paternal at the time, is what introduces desire and allows for an exit from the imaginary circuit at the lower level.

The prohibition of *jouissance* imposed by the Father is directly opposed to the premise of consumer capitalism, that which capitalizes on the superego's injunction to *enjoy* (Lacan, 1975/1998). The fissure here between the superego and the prohibiting Father highlights Lacan's differentiation between the ego ideal and the superego. The thrust, of course, is that it is no accident that consumer capitalism, with its will-to-*jouissance* as a "konstante Kraft" (Freud, 1915, p. 212), erodes the Father at every available opportunity while simultaneously pushing the subject to burnout in enjoyment (or perhaps burning up in consumption). To truly enjoy, the ego ideal—due to its regulatory function—must be overcome.

Indeed, Lacan (2011/2018) foresaw the problem brewing in society around the father; "*L'e-pater ne nous epate plus.* His wowing us is a thing of the past" (p. 184). Nonetheless, Lacan's optimism that something would always play the role of the father contrasts with some of his disciples, who view the time of the Father as over (see Miller, 2019).[2]

A point of clarification is necessary, however. Because the subject is an effect of discourse, some confusion may arise between whether what is involved in this change in discourse is necessarily a change in subjectivity. In other words, is a change in discourse something social or something individual? This calls to mind the disagreement between Freud's radical individualistic understanding of group formation and Durkheim's advocacy of a radical and ontologically weighty Social with a capital S. Lacan's elaboration of the subject as an effect of discourse places him, as Michelman (1996) proposed, in the position of a "bridge figure" between these traditions (p. 144); however, this does not clarify the question.

With respect to the individual and the social, the subject occupies a place at a nexus. This should be clear in Lacan's various graphs of desire as well as in the unnamed precursor of that graph at the start of *Formations of the Unconscious* (Lacan, 1998/2017a, p. 10). There are two intersecting lines in this precursor graph, one representing the signifying chain and the other, discourse. In this early form, discourse primarily refers to "the individual subject's concrete discourse," but Lacan was careful to state that this discourse is "discourse, such as is admitted into the code of the discourse that I will call the discourse of reality we all share" (p. 10). The code, which is the discourse of shared reality, Lacan went on immediately to clarify, is "located in the big Other" and that "it's absolutely necessary that this big Other exist" (p. 11). Lacan's later development that the big Other precisely does not exist does not negate the effects of the big Other that he cataloged at this stage of his seminar and continued to develop after his affirmation of the Other's nonexistence. The two lines intersect twice, with the individual subject's discourse passing through the signifying chain in a retroactive manner, passing between the code and the message, forming a circuit.

By the account in *Formations of the Unconscious*, discourse as shared occupies the place of the code within the individual subject's discourse, a point of intersection (Lacan, 1998/2017a). This is notable, as the subject is birthed in a particular discourse—its filial discourse—that renders possible the journey it treks in bisecting the signifying chain; at the same time, the discourse of the code contained in the Other may be distinct from the subject's filial discourse. This is most obvious when one learns a new language, but it also happens when one's native language changes. One might consider in the latter case the terms that are permitted or excluded from the discourse of an elder generation and that of the youngest within a given language group, at least for vibrant languages that continue to evolve. This means that the answer to the question of whether discourse is individual or social is, in one sense, both. The individual is birthed in a filial discourse and yet continues to move in a world governed by discourses that determine what signifiers are available to the subject. This reflects that there is also a disjunctive answer to the question of whether discourse is individual or social—aspects of the subject are always excluded from any discourse, which is why the subject is split from the beginning. The subject and discourse are mutually interdependent, then, even where they are exclusive.

Regarding the Freud-Durkheim distinction, Lacan (1998/2017a) made one more remarkable comment in this disquisition; after stating the necessity of the Other, Lacan argued that "there is absolutely no need to call it by the idiotic and delusional name 'collective consciousness'" (p. 11). This is seemingly a direct rebuke of Durkheim's sociological conception of an ontologically weighty society. For Lacan, the Other can inhabit even a solitary subject, such as the last speaker of a language. However, the rejection of Durkheim's collective consciousness is not a complete acceptance of a solely individualistic notion of psychic life. One is reminded of how, when Lacan (1973/1978) repudiated André Green's comment that Lacan was the "son of Hegel," Green responded by exclaiming that "the sons kill the father!" (p. 215). Perhaps his rejection of Durkheim is also somewhat overstated. Indeed, his comment about collective consciousness does nothing more than follow Freud's position, which it must be noted was not a complete rejection of the social aspects of psychic life. With respect to a different issue, that of the Jungian controversy, Freud (1939) noted, "I do not think we gain anything by introducing the concept of a 'collective' unconscious. The content of the unconscious, indeed, is in any case a collective, universal property of mankind," which, it is worth noting, Freud also connected to the acquisition of speech in early childhood (p. 132).

Because of the complex relationship between discourse and subjectivity, it is not enough to say that a new discourse—the fifth discourse—necessarily leads to new forms of subjectivity. It remains to be seen whether the effects of a new discourse actually produce a new subject or only new contours within the subjective structures that Lacan elaborated, which seems more likely. In other words, if lack is excluded in the fifth discourse, it does not by necessity follow that all subjects of this discourse are psychotic. The exclusion of lack or of desire in this discourse is not a foreclosure at the level of the subject; neither is it a repression or disavowal. Instead, it is a suppression—*Unterdrückung*. Lacan (1998/2017a) distinguished *Unterdrückung* from *Verdrängung* (repression) in a similar way as he distinguished Freud's ambiguous uses of ego ideal, ideal ego, and superego. Utilizing Freud's Signorelli parapraxis, Lacan clarified that *Unterdrückung* and *Verdrängung* occur at different levels and in different ways. What is *verdrängt* is kept in the level of the message-code circuit by the active force of repression; one retains the signifier within discourse, however much trouble there is in locating the signifier. In contrast, what is *unterdrückt* is lost from discourse, and such suppression "need happen but once and for all," where the signifier falls to a place beyond where the subject can reach. The signifier is not actively repressed because it is excluded from discourse. In this sense, lack is *unterdrückt* in the fifth discourse because it has fallen out of discourse altogether. Lack is not able to be heard or tolerated by the subject.

This is problematic for the social link. The fifth discourse's exclusion of lack is a breaking of boundaries, seeking to trample down regulation that could present a barrier to the freewheeling imaginary circuit. This means that symbolic identifications along traditional lines cannot be tolerated; this accelerated the decline of Americans' identifications with organized religion, but it also pushed against every identification prohibitive of indulgence. This included transforming the American identity from one defined by an ideal of rugged industriousness to one of cosmopolitan hedonism. Increasingly, the fifth discourse has also animated almost every aspect of public discourse in the US, from the corporations where it has long been at home to social media used by youth to the legal, social, and political issues that are reaching a fever pitch of polarization as a result of increasingly imaginary investments that suppress lack altogether. This is a combined erosion of integration and regulation, both of which stand in the way of maintaining a subject that is simultaneously in need and also never satisfied, without any recognition of desire.

Notes

1 I am basing this distinction in part on Soler's (2018) work, which I do not explicate here but do introduce more fully in Chapter 10.
2 Miller's (2019) "Fantasy" is another intriguing perspective with respect to the time after the Father. While I greatly respect Miller's work, I share Žižek's (2006) uncertainty about his formulation of the discourse of hypermodernity as the analyst's discourse.

References

Durkheim, É. (1979). *Suicide*. G. Simpson (Ed.). (J. A. Spaulding & G. Simpson, Trans.). Free Press. (Original work published 1897.)

Freud, S. (1915). Triebe und Triebschicksale. *Gesammelte Werker: Chronologisch Geordnet* (Vol. X), pp. 210–232.

Freud, S. (1921). Group psychology and the analysis of the ego. *The Standard Edition of the Complete Psychological Works of Sigmund Freud* (Vol. XVIII), pp. 65–144. Hogarth Press.

Freud, S. (1930). Civilization and its discontents. *The Standard Edition of the Complete Psychological Works of Sigmund Freud* (Vol. XXI), pp. 57–146. Hogarth Press.

Freud, S. (1939). Moses and monotheism: Three essays. *The Standard Edition of the Complete Psychological Works of Sigmund Freud* (Vol. XXIII), pp. 1–138. Hogarth Press.

Grigg, R. (n.d.). The concept of semblant in Lacan's teaching. *Lacan.com*. www.lacan.com/griggblog.html.

Lacan, J. (1968). From an Other to the other. (C. Gallagher, Trans.). Unpublished seminar. www.lacaninireland.com/web/wp-content/uploads/2010/06/Book-16-from-an-Other-to-the-other.pdf.

Lacan, J. (1971). On a discourse that might not be a semblance. (C. Gallagher, Trans.). Unpublished seminar. www.valas.fr/IMG/pdf/THE-SEMINAR-OF-JACQUES-LACAN-XVIII_d_un_discours.pdf.

Lacan, J. (1972). Du discours psychanalytique. (J. W. Stone, Trans.). https://freud2lacan.b-cdn.net/DISCOURSE_OF_CAPITALISM-bilingual.pdf.

Lacan, J. (1978). *The four fundamental concepts of psychoanalysis*. J. A. Miller (Ed.). (A. Sheridan, Trans.). W.W. Norton & Co. (Original work published 1973.)

Lacan, J. (1990). *Television: A challenge to the psychoanalytic establishment*. W. W. Norton & Co. (Original work published 1974.)

Lacan, J. (1998). *On feminine sexuality, the limits of love and knowledge*. J. A. Miller (Ed.). (B. Fink, Trans.). W.W. Norton & Co. (Original work published 1975.)

Lacan, J. (2007). *The other side of psychoanalysis*. J. A. Miller (Ed.). (R. Grigg, Trans.). W.W. Norton & Co. (Original work published 1991.)

Lacan, J. (2017a). *Formations of the Unconscious*. J. A. Miller (Ed.). (R. Grigg, Trans.). Polity. (Original work published 1998.)

Lacan, J. (2017b). *Talking to brick walls: A series of presentations in the chapel at Sainte-Anne Hospital*. J. A. Miller (Ed.) (A. R. Price, Trans.). Polity. (Original work published 2011.)

Lacan, J. (2018). *...Or worse*. J. A. Miller (Ed.) (A. R. Price, Trans.). Polity. (Original work published 2011.)

Michelman, S. (1996). Sociology before linguistics: Lacan's debt to Durkheim. In D. Pettigrew & F. Raffoul, *Disseminating Lacan* (pp. 123–150). State University of New York Press.

Miller, J. A. (2019). *Paradigms of jouissance: Three interventions by Jacques-Alain Miller*. (T. Sowley, M. Julien, J. Haney, & A. Duncan, Trans.). Psychoanalytical Notebooks.

Soler, C. (2018). *Humanisation? Psychoanalysis, symbolisation, and the body of the unconscious*. (B. Farrow & H. D'Alascio, Trans.). Routledge.

Stavrakakis, Y. (2007). *The Lacanian left: Psychoanalysis, theory, politics*. Edinburgh University Press.

Strachey, J. (1955). Editor's note before *Totem and Taboo*. In J. Strachey (Ed.), *The Standard Edition of the Complete Psychological Works of Sigmund Freud* (Vol. XIII), pp. ix–xi. Hogarth Press.

Vanheule, S. (2016). Capitalist discourse, subjectivity and Lacanian Psychoanalysis. *Frontiers in psychology*, 7. doi:10.3389/fpsyg.2016.01948.

Žižek, S. (2006). Jacques Lacan's four discourses. www.lacan.com/zizfour.htm.

6 A Broken Image
Technological Advancement and Youth Mental Health

The ludicrous celerity of technological advancement between the late 1990s to the early 2020s has placed the children of this generation at the inflection point of unprecedented social change, change even more potent in terms of its effects on the social link than that witnessed by the Greatest Generation, who were born in the time of horses and buggies and lived long enough to see the moon landing. When Freud (1930) was recounting the technological progress of his time, already remarkable as it was, he was keen to observe that such advancements in technology did not actually improve human happiness. Considering telephonic technology, telegrams, and medical advances, Freud trenchantly and, with palpable pessimism perhaps appropriate to his society at the time, observed that:

> If there had been no railway to conquer distances, my child would never have left his native town and I should need no telephone to hear his voice; if travelling [sic] across the ocean by ship had not been introduced, my friend would not have embarked on his sea-voyage and I should not need a cable to relieve my anxiety about him. What is the use of reducing infantile mortality when it is precisely that reduction which imposes the greatest restraint on us in the begetting of children, so that, taken all round, we nevertheless rear no more children than in the days before the reign of hygiene, while at the same time we have created difficult conditions for our sexual life in marriage, and have probably worked against the beneficial effects of natural selection? And, finally, what good to us is a long life if it is difficult and barren of joys, and if it is so full of misery that we can only welcome death as a deliverer?
>
> (p. 88)

That current advancements in technology, particularly the smartphone and social media, have similarly paradoxical effects is clear to even casual observers, including the adolescents who consume these services—or who are consumed by them. Rarely has there been a more farcically inapt phrase than "social media," whose giants profit precisely to the extent users are alone and absorbed not in those around them but in their devices. Who

DOI: 10.4324/9781032666334-9

would need a social network if one was actually connected to their community?

By putting the fingers of profit in all the interstices of human connection—from friendship, to ancestry, to romance, to sex, to sharing goods, to community—corporations have pried people apart, further and further. A corollary of this is that, once corporations gain control of these human connections, the connections are dislocated from the traditional nodes that once mediated them. Dislocated from nodes such as parents, teachers, religious leaders, parents of friends, or other such communal relations, digital connections are increasingly discrete and conducted outside the awareness of others in the local community of living beings, such as parents and siblings. This is a monumental shift in the social link; the integration and regulation of the link are no longer mediated first by the family and then by the local community in the same way as before.

With this transition in the social link follows a transition in rites of initiation. Traditionally, an initiation is conducted in a local community, in person, with credible community authorities. The novice's passage from family to community is known to and accepted by both the family and the community. The sexual knowledge received by the novice, which is implicated in both integration and regulation, is established within the social link in a way that is contiguous with the local community and the family. The smartphone—the Internet in the palm of one's hand—changed all of this. Most crucially, youth began to be immersed in exposures to a variety of cultures and social structures, with such exposures coming to place brackets around one's own local experience.

In constructing the significance of the change introduced by the increasingly connected world, *L'école Freudienne du Québec*—in particular Willy Apollon, Danielle Bergeron, and Lucie Cantin—have developed the idea of "world-formation," or *mondialisation*, which supplements the idea of *globalisation* in the French language (Librett, 2019). While *globalisation* refers more to the economic impact of what English calls globalization, *mondialisation* refers not only to this but to the broader impacts across societies of global exposure. World-formation, by blurring the boundaries of language and culture, entails a concomitant "world-*de*-formation" as well (p. 80). This de-formation of the world occurs because of the erosion of credibility of the social link and the social system. Librett (2019) elaborated:

> Given that language, like the social link it founds, is arbitrary…language (or the social link) always requires a supplementary guarantee of its meaningfulness and credibility. Belief—or faith—becomes crucial to the world of society in general, because we deal there with social representations, or semblances, which are not only always unfounded (society could always be constructed differently) but also alien and inadequate to the unsayable singularity of experience.
>
> (p. 85)

What can establish the belief in the system? "Narrative and symbolic attempts to shore up the authority of some transcendent Other who serves as a guarantor of the sustainability of the social order" (p. 86). In other words, a semblant of the Other, one we can make believe is capable of providing a guarantee. When this semblant dissolves, or when the group ceases to make use of it, the social link it supported collapses as well, and the drive energy that was bound in social covenants becomes unbound.

The transcendent Other, which animated the imperial cults and civil religions of societies past and sustains those in the present, is part of what becomes erased in world-formation. The rigor and violence that characterized the religious piety of the world for so long shows just how seriously humanity has taken the importance of behavioral synchrony, with almost every group in power taking steps to delimit or subordinate the heterodox beliefs of its others. Ultimately, the violence was not just about correct belief in itself, but about the necessity of a semblant for social organization. If another's god is just as valid as one's own, especially when they say different things, how can any god be trusted to hold the social order together? *Mondialisation* has led to an ongoing confrontation of the subject with other forms-of-life. When exposed in such a way, the subject can either respond by doubling down upon its semblant or release the semblant, with such release divesting the regulatory and identificatory bindings of *jouissance*.

Lacan (1998/2017) once described the Other as delivering a promissory note to the subject that might be redeemed at the coming of age. The exposure to other forms-of-life and other "gods" (ideologies, organizing principles, deities, governments, and so on) is a depreciation in such promissory notes, leading to a question of their validity to begin with. Although Lacan (1966/2006) eventually articulated a position different from his earlier one, stating that "there is no Other of the Other" (p. 688), the Other of the Other, as the semblant, still retains its power. As Laurent and Miller wrote about the Name of the Father, "one can only make do without the Name of the Father *qua* real on condition that one makes use of it as semblant" (as cited in Grigg, n.d.); in other words, the derealization of the Name of the Father only works if one retains it as a semblant. The subject and society will run into trouble functioning without such a semblant.

The exposure to the Internet, then, prompts the youth to question their filial discourse much earlier than in previous generations and with much greater frequency. Where a novice living anywhere in the 18th century might never have a significant encounter with another culture, for example, this is a virtual certainty today. This is especially complex as the Internet permits exposure to sexual knowledge to any user regardless of age and regardless of the filial discourse's narrative of the sexual difference or its navigation within the social link.

Amia Srinivasan (2021), a professor of social and political theory at Oxford University, wrote about her experiences discussing pornography with her students, who "were the first to have come of age sexually" in the

Internet age dominated by pornography (p. 41). In recounting a class discussion, she described how one female student inquired "if it weren't for pornography...how would we ever learn to have sex"? (p. 40). This sentiment is not restricted to this one person. One example of the role pornography plays in teaching sex is the fact that younger generations seem to consider choking during sex to be relatively routine in contrast to older generations, likely in part due to an increase in this sexual interaction being portrayed in pornography (Contos, 2022). Indeed, around 58 percent of undergraduate women reported having been choked during sex in one study (Herbenick et al., 2021).

Srinivasan's (2021) argument, in part, is that while "porn is not a pedagogy...it often functions as if it were" (p. 44). This is why another student came to her about her boyfriend complaining she was not having sex the "right" way, and Srinivasan called on a variety of research reflecting the position of authority that it occupies in young minds when it comes to sexual knowledge. In the United States, the erstwhile debate—still raging in some areas—about sex education reflects not simply a concern about the moral propriety of sex education in schools but also a conflict over who retains pedagogical rights: the family or society? Is it up to parents to decide when, how, and whether their children learn about sex? The irony is that while this conflict has been waged in the realm of public opinion, youth did not wait for the adults to decide who is in charge and took their questions to the oracle of porn. With all of this in mind, one might take a step further than Srinivasan and state that pornography is, in fact, a pedagogy of enjoyment.

Viola and Vorcaro (2018) also discussed the importance of sexual knowledge being transmitted in initiation rites, identifying this as a key feature of the rite. Typically, the education is given in the context of highly structured encounters between the novice and those conducting the initiation. When this is the case, the youth is tethered through the social references of the initiation, which Viola and Vorcaro argued connects the youth's body to the social body. In contrast to this contextualized induction into sexual knowledge is the access to limitless information available to youth through the Internet. This knowledge is, by and large, unregulated by the family or the local community, and it is not articulated within a coherent symbolic system such as local communities used to be able to construct or establish for the induction into knowledge. Rather, knowledge is not imparted by known adults to novice youth in a rite or through symbolic communication but incoherently through imaginary means—the "logic of the screen" (Srinivasan, 2021, p. 70). Even if an adolescent searches for practical information on sex through public health materials from a government or hospital system, this information is disconnected from any sense of meaning, community, or personal connection to the adolescent. Unfettered access to sexual knowledge often yields a traumatic *jouissance*, a horror-enjoyment, not simply with respect to pornography in its softcore forms but especially with respect to hardcore pornography, gore and films of death, and interactions with predatory o/Others. This access, once at least able to be mediated by familial observation of shared devices (e.g., the family computer in the living room) has become increasingly unmediated, with smartphones becoming increasingly ubiquitous and, except for the savviest of parents, difficult to monitor.

In the wake of the erosion of the social link from the disintegration of civil religion and the suppression of lack in consumerism, the Internet's role in delivering sexual knowledge to youth today has assumed the significance of the only reliable initiation rite. No matter how old or young the child is, they become an adult when they gain unfettered access to the Internet, with the whole host of human knowledge at their fingertips. Knowledge of the sexual difference and sexual rapport arrives without a symbolic structure already binding it—there is no discourse, of which the youth is already a subject, that assimilates it.[1]

Beyond direct exposure to pornography, unrestricted access to sexual knowledge is profuse in US culture generally. Consider the intersection of music and social media, such as Cardi B and Meghan Thee Stallion's (2020) song *WAP*,[2] tagged excerpts of which received more than 1.5 billion views on TikTok in one month (Rosenblatt, 2020). Indeed, among other accolades and recognitions, *WAP* topped the chart of the *Billboard* Global 200 for three (non-consecutive) weeks (Trust, 2020), which measures streaming and downloads across the globe; it was recognized by BBC News' analysis of best songs of 2020 as the best song of the year (Savage, 2020); and Meghan Thee Stallion and Cardi B performed this song live at 63rd annual Grammy Awards, resulting in more than 1,000 complaints to the Federal Communications Commissions (Shaffer, 2021).

WAP (Cardi B & Meghan Thee Stallion, 2020) manages to introduce listeners, in the course of three minutes and seven seconds, to *coitus interruptus* (the original Onanism), the importance of vaginal lubrication, cunnilingus, analingus, fellatio, deepthroat, public foreplay, sexual roleplay, bondage, the exchange of sexual favors for material goods, the importance of penile size and shape, and masochism. This highly dense song expresses sexual knowledge in a format freely available outside of local community contexts to anyone with Internet access. The effect of such a dissociation between sexual knowledge and societal regulation is a society in which youth, with greater technological instinct, have accordingly greater access to sexual knowledge than their parents. This phenomenon was humorously illustrated in a series of videos, produced primarily on TikTok, in which teenagers play *WAP* for their unsuspecting parents in order to video record their reactions (e.g., Trendy Tiktoks, 2020). Often, the teens laugh as their parents are variously scandalized or intrigued. But in every case, the parent is the one receiving the education; although the parent ostensibly has knowledge of sex (hence the child), the purity of the sexual enjoyment portrayed by *WAP*—which is completely absent any acknowledgment of sex's reproductive function outside of references to pulling out—is what provides the educative experience, wherein parents learn just what their children know. That this encounter of the parent with sexual knowledge is humorous reveals it to be a joke like any other, or perhaps an interpretation, and, indeed, interpretations often provoke laughter from the analysand (Freud, 1905, p. 170 footnote 1). Namely, it betrays the unconscious idea at its core: The parent has fallen from the position of the Other who regulates knowledge of sex.

The broader reality of the end of the transmission of sexual knowledge through social regulation in rites of initiation is testified to within *WAP* itself (Cardi B & Meghan Thee Stallion, 2020). Cardi B makes a quip in the song about macaroni, which is an ostensible reference to Mohammed Zoror's Vine (a video on the defunct social media platform of the same name, used for short videos) of 2016, in which he (then 16 years old) approaches his mother stirring a pot of macaroni and comments "that's what good pussy sounds like," and, similar to parental reactions to *WAP*, her reaction is the punchline (Zoror, 2014; Strapagiel, 2020).

The conservative outrage in response to *WAP* was predicated, supposedly, on the fear of conservatives about the effect of such music on children, such as Republican James P. Bradley's Twitter post regarding his fear and trembling for the future of children (Brown, 2020). Of course, Bradley's incredible claim to have heard the song "accidentally" is telling regarding his own relationship with such music. How does one accidentally listen to all three minutes of a song called *Wet-Ass Pussy*?

Of course, the other side of the conservative outrage is the *Wunsch*—fear and desire—for sexual enjoyment, betrayed by Bradley's "accidental" audition. Why hide the fact that one listened to such a song intentionally? Similarly, it is not novel to suggest an unconscious desire underlying the criticisms of, for example, Ben Shapiro, who couched his objections to *WAP* in part on a tongue-in-cheek concern for the sexual health of Cardi B and Meghan Thee Stallion. He noted his wife, a physician, stated such vigorous secretion of vaginal fluids is only achieved in pathological conditions (Shapiro, 2020). The aggressivity in relation to the other who has more enjoyment is not mysterious, and even the non-psychoanalytically minded Twitterati recognized this when they described Shapiro's concern as a "self-own" (Carlin, 2020). Even Shapiro's surprisingly catchy spoken-word rendition of the lyrics (of course remixed by others as a cover of the original) contained references only to "the P-word," the word *pussy* itself invested too greatly with *jouissance* to be born upon the tongue (cf. Mamo, 2020).

Obviously, there is a larger discussion—which occurred around the song's prominence—about the role of feminine *jouissance* in society and how men react to female enjoyment, and perhaps especially how white men react to black feminine enjoyment. This is a well-warranted discussion, particularly in light of the typically male-centered production of pornographic material providing formation of pubescent sexuality. While the consternation of Bradley and Shapiro seems to question the legitimacy of *WAP* (as a song or as a phenomenon), the concern regarding *WAP* here is not about the song itself but about the transition away from a cohesive and local contextualization of the sexual relationship and its effects on the social link.

The use of unregulated sexual knowledge as a method of demonstration, in which the subject confronts the Other (in the body of the parent) with the horror of the sexual knowledge it lacks, is critical in considering its relation to the unconscious. These demonstrations reveal less a perverse structure than a perverse moment in neurosis; perhaps a quasi-phobic reaction to produce the prohibitive Other due to precocious exposure to the sexual difference. In such cases, the subject is defending against the position of the object of *jouissance* for the Other, inducing in the Other a state of momentary confrontation with mental representations (*Vorstellungen*) connected to *jouissance*. Put another way, this refers the Other away from the subject and towards a different desire. That the subject should find itself in a place of questioning with relation to the Other—what am I to you?—is common, but the inability to produce an answer in the context of the social link is what makes this moment more perilous today. With respect to demonstration, what rendered the Shapiro "remix" of *WAP* (Harrison, 2020), with his dry reading of the lyrics laid over the original music, amusing to many is its incorporation of horror in the retelling; each use of "wet a P-word" embodies a confrontation with the horror of *jouissance* in the body of what has come to represent the Other for many—the conservative cishet white man. The listening subject itself finds *jouissance* in this weak censorship that impotently tries to reestablish a social regulation.

The music of another popular artist sheds further light upon this moment. Billie Eilish first began making music as a preteen, and first received significant attention around the age of 13 for her song *Ocean Eyes* (Eilish, 2015; Marsh, 2017). By 2021 her sophomore studio album, *Happier Than Ever*, was released to critical praise (Eilish, 2021a; BBC News, 2021). The first single from this album, *Oxytocin* (Eilish, 2021c), is significant for its aesthetic revisioning of God, who for millennia was the big Other whose name produced the initiation of the subject—in this sense, "God" is not only the Christian God, not only the Abrahamic God, but the God inclusive of these as well as the phallic deities at the head of various pantheons throughout history. The development of God's phallic masculinity as a defining feature as an elevation of an earthly father or fathers is notably challenged in *Oxytocin*, wherein God is feminized with she/her pronouns. Without tripping into a theological discussion, the use of feminine language for God presentifies the problem of the specular image as reflected in the God image—that is, the tendency of the powerful of humanity to make God in their own image (Lacan, 1986/1992). The use of feminine language does not introduce a new problem but reveals an old one, revealing that the construction of God in putatively symbolic terms covers over the imaginary constructions that typically underlie this (see Waitz & Tisdale, 2022).

Second, and more importantly, *Oxytocin* (Eilish, 2021c) imagines God in this song not only as a weak lawgiver (whose commands might be ignored based on the day of the week) but also as one who is overtaken by sexual excitement and indifference to her own rules, suggesting that she would be unable to resist engaging in a threesome with the singer[3] and the singer's sexual partner. This brings a very literal representation to Lacan's (1975/1998) identification of God as "the third party in this business of human love" (p. 70).

This catchy single is a representation of changes within society. Whereas in the past, God—especially the Abrahamic God—had occupied a position of symbolic authority in the United States, largely valuable from a sociological perspective for its role in providing behavioral synchrony and as a dead father whose prohibition could guarantee the order of society, the vision of God as a feminine subject engaged in a threesome shows the re-emergence of the other ancient vision of the Divine, the imaginary Divine, as seen in the gods of concupiscence, capable of *jouissance* and susceptible to sexual seduction. Importantly, this reflects less a change in theology than a change in the cosmology of the family system. The paternal no longer reliably causes fission, and the maternal does not always forswear the demand for *jouissance*.

This cosmological shift has many contributing factors. These include the larger deconstruction of founding narratives in the United States and the erasure of limits in consumerism, but technological advances have undeniably played a role in this as well, and not only in the sense of pornography or the sexual knowledge obtained in popular culture. The family has shifted away from a structure prioritizing a certain symbolic integration in a larger society along with a regulation that applies—and this is of crucial importance—to the parents as well as to the child. Instead, there is greater emphasis on the enjoyment of the parents, which serves to erase the limitations the child places on parental enjoyment as well as to model for the child how to properly become a consumer.

Among the most important technological advances enabling this change in family structure are the sophisticated and widely available forms of reproductive and family planning technologies. This might be traceable to the legalization of contraceptives such as condoms, which alter the conception of the child, who is no longer a "gift" from God but a biological accident of sex that may or may not be precluded. This is, in fact, a byproduct of the phenomenon Freud (1930) observed regarding reduced infant mortality: that increasing the likelihood of a child living to maturity increased the necessity of family planning. Separating sexual *jouissance* from reproduction—the former occurring in every case, the latter at certain moments—this technique implicitly privileges *jouissance* and throws the child into question. Furthermore, if the child is not a gift from God, the role of God becomes increasingly superfluous, as he is no longer needed for the appearance of a child. The narrative of how conception occurs is no longer "we conceived because we were supposed by God to conceive," but becomes "we conceived because we chose not to use a condom," or perhaps, "we shouldn't have conceived because we chose to use a condom." The explanatory models available no longer require an appeal to the Other.

The 1965 *Griswold v. Connecticut* decision of the Supreme Court of the United States established the privacy element of the Constitution and the right of married couples to make their own decisions regarding contraceptive use without interference from the state. There is no coincidence that this ruling paved the way for the legalization of abortion on the same grounds of privacy (until *Dobbs v. Jackson Women's Health Organization* [2021]), further moving procreation from the realm of the social to the private and individual. Contemporary scientific advancements established *in vitro* fertilization and the freezing of eggs as options for those planning to become parents. These legal and technological advances represent a previously unimaginable shift in the traditional and historical fabric of society; they mark a sliding of *jouissance* under reproduction, reinforced all along by the increasing prominence of pornography and pornographization as further elements of sexual *jouissance* beyond reproduction.

The relevance of these matters to the child is that the new narrative of the child's conception no longer creates a duty owed by the parents to the Other—to God, to society, to community, and so on. This puts the child's role in question with respect to the parents and society, a precarious position wherein the purpose of the child outside the family is not readily apparent and conflation of the child with the object is more easily retained. As Freud (1930) observed, families are reluctant to surrender their children to the Other, which is all the more true when the Other is not accessible.

The legal and technological advances making a range of reproductive decisions possible are important, and the fallout from *Dobbs v. Jackson Women's Health Organization* reveals the consequences that rolling back these advances would have. One challenge for the psychoanalyst is appraising things as they are rather than arguing for how they ought to be. In this case, there are very real societal and libidinal consequences to these legal and technological advances in human reproduction, even if we do not want them to go away. Beyond the immediate questions of choice and privacy, there is the profound demarcation point between the ways of humanity before and after the 20th century. The Catholic Church's ancient positions with respect to contraception and abortion are horrifying to many in part because they assume a castration to which U.S. society (and technologically advanced societies generally) has grown unaccustomed—that purity of enjoyment is not the reality of life after all. As Anne-Marie Cummins (2023) put it, "no longer is having children a contribution to the 'common weal': no longer is it a social duty or a necessity—it is a personal and private choice undertaken in the expectation of existential fulfillment" (p. 97). What she casts as a child's emotional labor on behalf of the parent can, in Lacanian terms, be understood as the parents' refusal of lack, which is apparent in Cummins' appeal to the characterization of Gherovici and Webster (2014) of certain forms of parenting as seeking to eliminate desire altogether.

To be clear, I do not advocate that the government curtail personal freedoms. One thing that has become all too clear in recent years is that there is little room in public discourse for nuanced considerations of important and complex topics; my hope is that academic literature is one space wherein such complexities can be faced without fear of collapse. If psychoanalysts are willing to consider the effects of capitalism on society, we must not overlook the effects of capitalism on the family, when children become another product—one should not forget that one IVF cycle can cost $30,000 (Conrad & Grifo, 2023). In consumerism, the choice to conceive becomes commodified like everything else—and to conceive becomes a choice of *jouissance*. There is no question more revealing of one's *Weltanschauung* than why one conceived a child—one's religion or economics hold no candle to this question. This isn't to say all conception has become about *jouissance* but that old narratives around childbirth have become degraded like old audiotapes, no longer playing back with the same clarity and giving only the impression of a nostalgia attached to a time quaint and backward compared with today.

If castration is absent in the parents' consumerist dream of completion and the child is conceived in the context of the parents' *jouissance* (i.e., for the parents to enjoy), it becomes difficult to envisage God in any other way than as a maternal Other who crosses the incest taboo, indulging in a *menage-à-trois* with her children. This is perhaps more a pleasant idea than the notion of an angry paternal God who enjoys the suffering of his creation in eternal conscious torment, although structurally the two are similar—God creates humans to produce its own *jouissance*; this is humanity's "chief end" (Westminster Assembly, 1647, §1). In fact, knowledge of *jouissance* is ultimately what animates the demonstrations of adolescents. Those who play songs like *WAP* for their parents or who define for them what "good pussy" sounds like are not demonstrating a knowledge of anatomical sex but a knowledge of *jouissance*. The youth are sharing with the parent that *they know where they came from*.

The production of children as containers of parental *jouissance* influences the child, whether from the parents' living vicariously through the child (which is different from high expectations) or from the parents' direct use of the child. In the current hypermodern moment, the attributes of the child are assumed over its actual presence in the world, the equivalent of the iconography of a floppy disk signifying a save function. The skeuomorphic origin becomes lost; the separation of *the parent's mental representation of the child* from *the child* collapses or does not occur consistently. The child is still the child, but its significance has shifted underneath it from *symbolic phallus* to *imaginary phallus*. This results in the construction, for the child, only of the little other, and not sufficiently of the big Other.

This consequently means, first, that the incest taboo has not been fully instantiated and not supported at a societal level, and second, that the shift of identification from the family to society is orders of magnitude more difficult to effect. The growing "failure to launch" phenomenon, which is not reducible to economic pressures, is perhaps the most colloquially familiar consequence of this slip, followed closely by the notion of adulting, that is, to play the adult or make-believe adulthood. Adulthood, the other side of initiation, is only a mirage for many younger folks today, a status which one can only mimic with more or less verisimilitude to the imagined ideal.

Carrying forward the hypermodern shift from symbolic to imaginary, whereas the rite of passage provides a symbolic identification—a new name, a role, or identity for the subject in the social link—the world of the specular image, dominated by pornography, music videos, and social media, provides instead an imaginary identification. Thus, instead of facilitating the navigation of the subject through the movement from family to society, these imaginary media—perhaps especially social media—illuminate the mirror as though it were the social link itself; instead of a naming Other, there is an impersonal algorithm. In this world, virtual interaction becomes everything. Social media prioritizes the engagement of the subject in the medium. In order to promote engagement and interaction, the algorithm determines the best way to provoke the subject. One prominent method is through feeding the subject politically inflammatory rhetoric (Merrill & Oremus, 2021; Munn, 2020). This is the well-documented approach of Meta, which stoked the flames of division throughout the term of President Trump, culminating in the *putsch* of January 6, 2021. This targeted use of the splintering of the social link to increase profits occurs at the intersection of political ideology, consumer capitalism, and hypermodernism.

Similarly, social media—Meta again holding the place of prominence, although Snap and ByteDance are not far behind—extend for youth the perfect mirror image (Wells et al., 2021). The use of Instagram by young girls has actively contributed to serious problems, including the acquisition of eating disorders. While some use social media in a passive fashion, others who actively participate strive to be the object for a massive audience of strangers. Whether this is the object of *jouissance* or a form of an hysterical embodiment of the object of desire varies, but the presentation is largely similar. The subject dresses, behaves, stages interactions, or livestreams their intimate moments for the enjoyment of the other, the gaze presentified in the form of the quantity of views, number of interactions, or accounts viewing a stream. Of course, under the predominance of the image, sexualization is the capitalist route of greatest efficiency (along with inflaming emotional tensions) for securing promotion in the algorithms of social media. If more people like images of the subject's body, then their following is increased, their account is promoted by the platform, and the subject is liable to receive promotional contacts for advertising products by adorning their body with them.

More interactions on a given social network mean more eyes watching it, which means either or both more advertising dollars or more metadata to sell. In either case, social media has a vested interest in providing compensation to prominent or successful social media users, or influencers. People of all ages are paid by social media companies (Dellatto, 2022) and third parties (Lieber, 2018) to produce content that garners interaction, thus either supporting the use of the platform directly or modeling the desirability of a consumer product. By reinforcing the use of the body as an economic object, this process promotes the ideal body ego increasingly replacing the ego ideal as the agency governing the social link. Hence the significance of youth—especially but not only females—feeling low self-worth after scrolling through social media; if the ideal ego governs the social link and a young person perceives themselves as not able to compete at the imaginary level, dysphoria will follow.

The objectification of the body turns mainstream social media platforms into pseudopornographic ones, where even youth produce sexually suggestive images of themselves to be desired or enjoyed by others (Levine, 2022). This goes beyond mildly suggestive selfies, with livestreams on TikTok in which viewers request specific acts from the (usually young, female) subject in exchange for specific monetary compensation, such as showing feet or taking off layers of clothes. The consonance between this and adult entertainment streams seem quantitative rather than qualitative; in fact, OnlyFans and TikTok have developed into a "symbiotic relationship" with one another (Carman, 2020, para. 4). While some content creators on OnlyFans use TikTok essentially for marketing purposes, it also happens that some who create TikTok accounts are asked so frequently whether they have an OnlyFans account that they go on to create them. This symbiotic relationship implicates minor adolescents, who may see content from sex workers promoting their OnlyFans pages on TikTok. TikTok, for its part, bans sexual content, yet its algorithm promotes the popular content of these users to broad audiences, and it is left up to the content creators to try to keep minor users from interacting with their content. This is a tall task for those with a large number of followers.

The sexualizing pressure of the anonymous Internet on young women and girls is also revealed in specific cases as well. Millie Bobby Brown, for example, came to fame prior to reaching adulthood. She was the target of a Reddit group counting down to her 18th birthday and saw increasingly sexualizing interaction from Internet users with her social media around the same time (Soteriou, 2022), and she is far from the first to be exposed to such pressures.

Indeed, the public image of Billie Eilish serves as a remarkable condensation of these societal developments. Eilish spent her adolescence in the public eye, and became well known for her fashion sense, which typically included bulky clothes, sports shorts, puffy jackets, and other articles that obscured her physical form (Xidias, 2019). This became iconic enough to spur discussion of her fashion sense and inspire other artists' music (e.g., Armani White, 2022). These clothes, Eilish later disclosed, were an effort to avoid judgment of her body (Xidias, 2019); here, Lacan's (1973/1978) play between *separare, se parare, se parer,* and *se parere* in his *Four Fundamental Concepts of Psychoanalysis* is brought to life by the clothing with which Eilish adorned herself. The obstruction of the gaze with obfuscatory clothing provides a separation from the Other that is not effected in a social link predicated on the imaginary.

Once she turned 18, Eilish (2020) addressed the issue of the Other's view of her body in a performance piece titled *Not My Responsibility*, a spoken word vocal performance accompanied by a video of her removing layers of clothing. Eilish's (2020) observation, in brief, was how public sentiment about her changes based on her wardrobe, recapitulating the so-called Madonna-Whore dynamic Freud (1912) set out in his work on the debasement of women common in the sphere of love. This is, for Eilish (2020), coupled with the gaze with which she has grown up.

While it is tempting to characterize Eilish's experience as nothing more than yet another repetition of the masculine gaze (which influences men and women alike) without substantive advancement from Freud's time, it would be a mistake to do so for the precise reason that the Internet reflects a monumental shift from this earlier era. With its quasi-anonymity, emphasis on the image, and removal from the reality of day-to-day life, it seems that the male gaze of the Internet prefers the "whore." Perhaps the Madonna continues to exist in some real life relationships and in the idealizations of women on the Internet, not unlike the courtly love Lacan (1986/1992) analyzed. Nevertheless, the fact that girls on social media and the Internet are, prior to their majority, subjected to age countdowns, encouraged to create adult streaming accounts, and sexualized with monetary compensation should clearly illustrate the way in which the Internet has changed the social landscape since Freud's time, particularly in its formation of young persons' identities, regardless of sex. Increasingly, the debasement does not occur between a man and a woman in the context of intimate relations but— thanks to social media—it has been democratized.

Eilish (2021b), on the same album as *Oxytocin* and *Not My Responsibility*, included the title track *Happier Than Ever*, which elaborates the singer's experience of a romantic relationship. At around five minutes, it is among Eilish's longest productions. The first half of the song is relatively characteristic for Eilish's style, containing mild acoustic instrumentation and soft, gentle vocals "that wouldn't have sounded out of place at a jazz club 60 years ago" (Thompson, 2021, para. 1). The singer considers her ambivalence, doubt, and realization that she is happiest when not around her partner. Around halfway through the song, however, the tone of the music changes, the instrumentation becomes more agitated, and by the end, Eilish is screaming "fuck you" over distorted electric guitar riffs that sound more typical of the emo punk of the early 2000s than the rest of her body of work.

To discuss this song is not a mere diversion into cultural critique, but an observation of a truth about the social link contained within the pinnacle of pop music at a certain moment in time. In this song, Eilish (2021b) may not necessarily have been writing from a fictional perspective but actually addressing her relationship with rapper Brandon Adams (Chow, 2021). Eilish was 16 when the relationship started, while Adams was five years older than her (Twersky, 2021). Eilish (2021b) makes ostensible reference to their age difference in *Happier Than Ever*, referring to herself in the second half of the song as a kid, suggesting a naivete which the Other has exploited. Indeed, several of Eilish's songs on this album include references to masculine abuse. The cut in the middle of the track *Happier Than Ever* that splits the two sides of the song is a moment of understanding. In the first half of the song, the Eilish's dulcet tones hem and haw, expressing a lack of clarity, confusion, and engaging interrogatively with the partner, inquiring about their intentions. The non-vocally expressed moment of realization moves the song into the more aggressive calling-to-account that composes the rest of the song. This silent realization is the moment of initiation, passage from childhood to adulthood, such that Eilish, after the moment, can refer to herself as a kid in the time before.

The significance of this is twofold. First, the initiation is completely elided from the vocal expression in the song, and even at an instrumental level, it is nothing other than a beat of rest and a change in tempo. This elision reflects the lack of inclusion in discourse of an initiation into adulthood. Second, the structure of the song also indicates that the initiation rite, such as it is able to function credibly in the US today, is a *deferred action* (Freud, 1950). One realizes one has crossed the threshold only after the fact, in contrast to the initiation rites of generations past when a debut or ritual might be anticipated and constructed prospectively as a moment to which one might look forward. This initiation by deferred action reflects the *ad hoc* nature of initiation rites in the US today. When an occasion presents itself, unfortunately often in the form of trauma, the novice is confronted with the significance of sexuality in their own subjective structure. When this sexual knowledge is delivered outside of local communities and symbolic contexts, it is much more likely to be overwhelming, unbound, and traumatic, however it appears. Thus, the failure of initiation rites renders the second phase of the biphasic sexuality of the human as traumatic, as *jouissance* is not bound and regulated and the youth is faced with the injunction only to enjoy it. When youth discover this *jouissance*, it is often either as something hidden and unexplained or as explained only by the Other without limits who says to enjoy.

Jerry Mander wrote in 1977 that "we humans slowly turn into whatever images we carry in our minds" (p. 216). The power of the image in social media far exceeds the power Mander worried about with respect to the television. The loss of the natural environment and the mode of experience to which humanity was so long accustomed have likewise accelerated, to the point we can no longer trust our senses due to the rapid development of artificial intelligence. The imaginary has increasingly flattened our society and kept youth from being able to enter the social link as historically constructed.

Youth are not left without recourse to some form of initiation, however. Speaking beings have always found a pathway forward. Today, youth at times have made use of *ad hoc* initiations in the form of deferred action noted above; others have done work to cobble together resolutions to the failure of initiation into the social link and adulthood, sometimes completely on their own, sometimes with help. The most frequent resolutions are the subject of the next part of this book.

Notes

1 One might argue that pornography or sexual knowledge on the Internet certainly can be contextualized in a discourse; this is partially true. In one sense, it might be true that a societal discourse may include pornography in through approval or opprobrium regarding its use, but the actual content of the pornography itself is not generally delivered as part of such a discourse, meaning this knowledge is dislocated and out of place. Of course, part of Srinivasan's (2021) argument is that pornography itself is a discourse, which is true in the sense she argues it, although from a Lacanian perspective, some nuance would be needed to distinguish between the way in which some pornography may reinforce certain forms of the master's or hysteric's discourses and the way in which it structures itself according to the imaginary and all this implies for the subject's assumption of it as knowledge.
2 For those unfamiliar, WAP stands for "Wet-Ass Pussy." I should be clear that the discussion of this song is not a criticism of the song or the artists. My point is that youth have relatively unfiltered access to sexually explicit music that is detailed enough to be considered a conduit of sexual knowledge.
3 I use "singer" rather than Eilish's name, just as the narrator in a book is not necessarily the same as the author. Eilish is known for her music's diverse vantage points, such as a song performed from the perspective of a serial killer (Barlow, 2017).

References

Armani White. (2022). Billie Eilish [song]. On *Road to CASABLANCO*. Legend-bound; Def Jam Recordings.

Barlow, E. (2017, February 24). Billie Eilish's "Bellyache" is totally psycho and per-fectly pop. *Vice*. www.vice.com/en/article/9a8xja/billie-eilishs-bellyache-is-tota lly-psycho-and-perfectly-pop.

Brown, A. (2020, August 7). California congressional candidate slams Cardi B and Megan Thee Stallion's 'WAP'. *LA Times*. www.latimes.com/entertainment-arts/m usic/story/2020-08-07/cardi-b-megan-thee-stallion-wap-congressional-candidate-j ames-bradley.

Cardi B & Megan Thee Stallion. (2020). WAP [song]. On *WAP*. Atlantic.

Carlin, B. W. (2020, August 10). Ben Shapiro self-owning himself by admitting he doesn't get his wife wet is excellent content [image attached] [post]. *X*. https://twitter.com/BaileyCarlin/status/1292940132455251969?lang=en.

Carman, A. (2020, September 17). OnlyFans stars say TikTok is making them rich. *The Verge*. www.theverge.com/2020/9/17/21439657/onlyfans-tiktok-subscribers-videos-fans.

Chow, A. R. (2021, July 30). 4 takeaways from Billie Eilish's new album Happier Than Ever. *Time*. https://time.com/6086022/billie-eilish-happier-than-ever.

Conrad, M. & Grifo, J. (2023, August 14). How much does IVF cost? *Forbes Health*. www.forbes.com/health/womens-health/how-much-does-ivf-cost/.

Contos, C. (2022, December 7). Sexual choking is now so common that many young people don't think it even requires consent. *The Guardian*. www.theguardian.com/commentisfree/2022/dec/08/sexual-choking-is-now-so-common-that-many-young-people-dont-think-it-even-requires-consent-thats-a-problem.

Cummins, A. M. (2023). "I love you more": Making childing visible–children's emotional labor in affluent libidinal economies. In M. O'Loughlin, C. Owens, & L. Rothschild (Eds), *Precarities of 21st century childhoods: Critical explorations of time(s), place(s), and identities*, pp. 95–108. Lexington Books.

Dellatto, M. (2022, May 5). TikTok will share ad revenue with some creators. *Forbes*. www.forbes.com/sites/marisadellatto/2022/05/04/tiktok-will-share-ad-revenue-with-some-creators.

BBC News. (2021, July 30). Billie Eilish: Critics praise 'defiant' second album, Happier Than Ever. www.bbc.com/news/entertainment-arts-58024655.

Dobbs v. Jackson Women's Health Organization. 597 U.S. 215 (2022). www.supremecourt.gov/opinions/21pdf/597us1r58_gebh.pdf.

Eilish, B. (2015). Ocean eyes [song]. SoundCloud. https://soundcloud.com/billieeilish/ocean-eyes.

Eilish, B. (2020). Not my responsibility [video]. YouTube. https://youtu.be/ZlvfYmfefSI.

Eilish, B. (2021a). Happier than ever [album]. Darkroom; Interscope.

Eilish, B. (2021b). Happier than ever [song]. On *Happier than ever*. Darkroom; Interscope.

Eilish, B. (2021c). Oxytocin [song]. On *Happier than ever*. Darkroom; Interscope.

Freud, S. (1905). Jokes and their relation to the unconscious. *The Standard Edition of the Complete Psychological Works of Sigmund Freud* (Vol. VIII), pp. 1–247. Hogarth Press.

Freud, S. (1912). On the universal tendency to debasement in the sphere of love. *The Standard Edition of the Complete Psychological Works of Sigmund Freud* (Vol. XI), pp. 177–190. Hogarth Press.

Freud, S. (1930). Civilization and its discontents. *The Standard Edition of the Complete Psychological Works of Sigmund Freud* (Vol. XXI), pp. 57–146. Hogarth Press.

Freud, S. (1950). Project for a scientific psychology. *The Standard Edition of the Complete Psychological Works of Sigmund Freud* (Vol. I), pp. 281–391. Hogarth Press.

Gherovici, P. & Webster, J. (2014). Observations from working with female obsessionals. *European Journal of Psychoanalysis*, 1(2), np. www.journal-psychoanalysis.eu/articles/observations-from-working-with-female-obsessionals.

Grigg, R. (n.d.). The concept of semblant in Lacan's teaching. *Lacan.com*. www.lacan.com/griggblog.html.

Griswold v. Connecticut. 381 U.S. 479 (1965). www.loc.gov/item/usrep381479.

Harrison, E. (2020, August 12). Ben Shapiro's criticism of Cardi B and Megan Thee Stallion's 'WAP' made into remix. *The Independent*. www.independent.co.uk/a

rts-entertainment/music/news/cardi-b-megan-thee-stallion-ben-shapiro-wap-remix
-a9667551.html.

Herbenick, D., Patterson, C., Beckmeyer, J., Gonzalez, Y. R. R., Luetke, M., Guerra-Reyes, L., Eastman-Mueller, H., Valdivia, D. S., & Rosenberg, M. (2021). Diverse ssexual behaviors in undergraduate students: Findings from a campus probability survey. *Journal of Sexual Medicine*, 18(6), 1024–1041. doi:10.1016/j.jsxm.2021.03.006.

Lacan, J. (1978). *The four fundamental concepts of psychoanalysis*. J. A. Miller (Ed.). (A. Sheridan, Trans.). W.W. Norton & Co. (Original work published 1973.)

Lacan, J. (1992). *The ethics of psychoanalysis*. J. A. Miller (Ed.). (R. Grigg, Trans.). W. W. Norton & Co. (Original work 1986.)

Lacan, J. (1998). *On feminine sexuality, the limits of love and knowledge*. J. A. Miller (Ed.). (B. Fink, Trans.). W.W. Norton & Co. (Original work published 1975.)

Lacan, J. (2006). *Ecrits*. (B. Fink, Trans.). W.W. Norton & Co. (Original work published 1966.)

Lacan, J. (2017). *Formations of the Unconscious*. Polity. (Original work published 1998.)

Levine, A. S. (2022, April 27). How TikTok live became a "strip club filled with 15-year-olds." *Forbes*. www.forbes.com/sites/alexandralevine/2022/04/27/how-tiktok-live-became-a-strip-club-filled-with-15-year-olds/?sh=531e8df962d7.

Librett, J. S. (2019). The subject in the age of world-formation (mondialisation): Advances in Lacanian theory from the Québec Group. In A. Govrin & J. Mills (Eds), *Innovations in psychoanalysis*, pp. 75–99. Routledge.

Lieber, C. (2018, November 28). How and why do influencers make so much money? The head of an influencer agency explains. *Vox*. www.vox.com/the-goods/2018/11/28/18116875/influencer-marketing-social-media-engagement-instagram-youtube.

Mamo, H. (2020, August 10). Ben Shapiro reads the censored lyrics to Cardi B and Megan Thee Stallion's 'WAP' & he can't handle it. *Billboard*. www.billboard.com/music/rb-hip-hop/ben-shapiro-reads-censored-wap-lyrics-cardi-b-megan-thee-stallion-9432034.

Mander, J. (1977). *Four arguments for the elimination of television*. Perennial.

Marsh, A. (2017, Feb 24). How Billie Eilish's "Ocean Eyes" turned her into an overnight sensation. *Teen Vogue*. www.teenvogue.com/story/how-billie-eilishs-ocean-eyes-turned-her-into-an-overnight-sensation.

Merrill, J. B. & Oremus, W. (2021, October 6). Five points for anger, one for a 'like': How Facebook's formula fostered rage and misinformation. *The Washington Post*. www.washingtonpost.com/technology/2021/10/26/facebook-angry-emoji-algorithm.

Munn, L. (2020). Angry by design: toxic communication and technical architectures. *Humanities and Social Sciences Communications*, 7, article no. 53. doi:10.1057/s41599-020-00550-7.

Rosenblatt, K. (2020, September 6). Cardi B shared this choreographer's 'WAP' dance. *NBC News*. www.nbcnews.com/pop-culture/viral/cardi-b-shared-choreographer-s-wap-dance-then-it-went-n1239446.

Savage, S. (2020, December 21). The best albums and songs of 2020: Fiona Apple, Cardi B, Bob Dylan and Dua Lipa. *BBC News*. www.bbc.com/news/entertainment-arts-55336503.

Shaffer, C. (2021, April 13). The FCC received over 1,000 complaints for Grammys 'WAP' performance. *Rolling Stone*. www.rollingstone.com/music/music-news/cardi-b-megan-thee-stallion-wap-performance-grammys-fcc-complaints-1155254/.

Shapiro, B. (2020, August 10). As I also discussed on the show, my only real concern is that the women involved—who apparently require a [post]. *X*. https://twitter.com/benshapiro/status/1292927011724304384?lang=en.

Soteriou, S. (2022, February 21). The reaction to Millie Bobby Brown's 18th birthday has sparked a discussion about the sexualization of female child stars after Emma Watson and Natalie Portman shared their similar experiences. *BuzzFeed*. www.buzzfeednews.com/article/stephaniesoteriou/millie-bobby-brown-18th-birthday-creepy-sexualized-child.

Srinivasan, A. (2021). *The right to sex: Feminism in the twenty-first century*. Farrar, Straus and Giroux.

Strapagiel, L. (2020, August 13). "WAP" has given new life to this iconic Vine about what macaroni and cheese sounds like. *Buzzfeed*. www.buzzfeednews.com/article/laurenstrapagiel/iconic-good-pussy-vine-inspired-wap.

Thompson, S. (2021, July 30). Billie Eilish, 'Happier Than Ever'. *NPR*. www.npr.org/sections/now-playing/2021/07/30/1022869253/billie-eilish-happier-than-ever.

Trendy Tiktoks. (2020, September 1). PARENTS REACT TO WAP TIKTOK COMPILATION [video]. *YouTube*. https://youtu.be/oq8RjfkjFkU?si=DzINfLDTpWWxt5vF.

Trust, G. (2020, October 5). Cardi B & Megan Thee Stallion's 'WAP' and BTS' 'Dynamite' lead latest Billboard Global Charts. *Billboard*. www.billboard.com/pro/cardi-b-wap-bts-dynamite-lead-latest-global-charts.

Twersky, C. (2021, April 29). Here are all the facts on Billie Eilish's former secret boyfriend, Q. *Seventeen*. www.seventeen.com/celebrity/celebrity-couples/a35645667/billie-eilish-ex-boyfriend-q-brandon-adams.

Viola, D. T. D. & Vorcaro, Â. M. R. (2018). A adolescência em perspectiva: Um exame da variabilidade da passagem à idade adulta entre diferentes sociedades. *Psicologia, Teoria e Pesquisa*, 34. doi:10.1590/0102.3772e3448.

Waitz, C & Tisdale, T. C. (2022). *Lacanian Psychoanalysis and Eastern Orthodox Christian Anthropology in Dialogue*. Routledge.

Wells, G., Horwitz, J. & Seetharaman, D. (2021, September 14). Facebook knows Instagram is toxic for teen girls, company documents show. *The Wall Street Journal*. www.wsj.com/articles/facebook-knows-instagram-is-toxic-for-teen-girls-company-documents-show-11631620739?mod=hp_lead_pos7&mod=article_inline.

Westminster Assembly. (1647). Westminster Shorter Catechism.

Xidias, A. (2019, June 25). Billie Eilish on her love of fashion and why she opts for oversized styles. *Vogue*. www.vogue.com.au/celebrity/interviews/billie-eilish-on-her-love-of-fashion-and-why-she-opts-for-oversized-styles/news-story/c45786b69c9979a75f69c58ee66e728d.

Zoror, M. (2014, December 31). Untitled [video]. *Vine*. https://vine.co/v/OwHOuZpu5Dw.

Part III
Le Mal de la Jeunesse

7   The Murder of Agamemnon

Introduction

The consequences of the erosion of initiation rites in the United States are becoming increasingly apparent. I am uncertain as to whether the rise of the consumerist fifth discourse marks an entry into a new epoch of subjectivity. Even after his Milan lecture on May 12, 1972, when Lacan suggested the master's discourse was being substituted by the capitalist discourse, he stated (only a little over a month later) that "the discourse of the master was the first to arise, and this is the discourse that has endured and which stands little chance of being shaken" (Lacan, 2011/ 2018, pp. 203–204). He also argued that the existence of the One, under which he categorized "everything that has so far been said about *Totem and Taboo*" (p. 179), was necessary because "we can say absolutely nothing that resembles anything that might constitute a truth function if we do not admit the necessity of *there being at-least-one who says no*" (p. 184). The negation of the Other is a necessary component of truth. He noted that this paternal function would operate without "flesh and blood" if needed (p. 184), and that castration is a logical necessity for language to obtain. Given Lacan's clarity on this matter, it may be early yet to determine whether new subjectivities exist. Nonetheless, the new symptoms analysts have been talking and writing about must have some origin. I will argue that there may be some innovation in subjectivity without necessarily conceding a widespread shift in the field of subjectivity as a result of late-stage capitalism.

The changes in the social link and discourse that apparently cause the new symptoms are intimately connected with the loss of initiation rites. As a review of the arguments regarding initiation rites thus far, one might define the rite of initiation as an embodied act that:

1   Marks an identification or naming that governs entrance into the social link.
2   Binds and names the pubertal upsurge in *jouissance* in the social link through the intervention of social knowledge.

DOI: 10.4324/9781032666334-11

These two elements both contain a reference to naming. Although I have generally, up to now, referred to the process of initiation as a reinforcement of the paternal function established in childhood, this is a slight over-simplification. Guerra (2020) considered the moment of adolescence to call for something beyond the paternal function, specifically a nomination capable of intervening not only in the symbolic but also in the real. The Name-of-the-Father, as a symbolic interdiction, establishes the identification with the ego ideal and the unary trait, providing a symbolic name. However, a real nomination must also bind the real—including a real *jouissance*—in such a way that it is accounted for within the social link. This is important, as the real of *jouissance* is a primary issue in the lives of youth today.

The overriding result of the disappearance of such a naming that can bind the symbolic and real for youth is two-fold: first, a degeneration of local communities, owing to a lack of shared identification, and second, an upsurge in *jouissance* that is unbound and unbindable within the confines of the fifth discourse. These two consequences are not separable and coincidental; the unbound *jouissance* is a consequence of the loss of the social link. However, these are only the formal consequences. The fallout travels further.

With generations growing up without induction into the social link, it should come as no surprise that the social link is deteriorating to a danger-ous degree. The social link is not so much dissipating—such that it would disappear for those already initiated—but dying, falling far below the repla-cement rate for a stable community. The crisis of youth is already the crisis of the entire body politic, and there is an undeniable connection between the geometric political polarization occurring in the US and the mental illness of youth.

Furthermore, the phenomena that are increasingly present in young per-sons are, once one has the conceptual framework of a Freudian-Lacanian initiation rite, easily explicable. I have referenced the mystery of adulting twice in this regard, along with the parallel problem of a "failure to launch," and these could be what else other than a failure of initiation? The family retains the child.

The responses of contemporary youth to the absence of initiation rites seem to fall along three pathways, affected by their own attractors. This excludes a fourth group, a group that is largely consistent with previous generations and who, through some filial discourse or extant local community, have retained an initiation into the social link capable of sustaining subjectivity without instability. With respect to those without such recourse, the first group is characterized by wild attempts to domesticate *jouissance*, faltering through a new world all alone. The second and third groups resolve the issue of *jouissance* not so much with wild attempts but with binding *jouissance* in substitute initiations.

The idea of "substitute initiations" is something of a parallel to Freud's (1930) "substitutive satisfactions" (p. 108). If it is satisfactory, how is it a substitute? Lacan (1973/1978) pulled on this same thread, pointing out that Freud's notion of satisfaction as attaining the aim of the drive is paradoxical if aim-inhibited satisfaction is also a possibility, as in sublimation. In this case, if something achieves the act of initiation, how is it a substitute initiation? While substitutive satisfactions have to do with the thoroughly sexual nature of the unconscious, calling an initiation a "substitute" here refers to two matters. First, it is a reference to the way in which the substitute initiations exchange the ego ideal for the ideal ego—the symbolic for the imaginary. Second, it also references that, in the past, initiation rites typically belonged to a certain locally identifiable people or community; increasingly these rites are voluntaristic and disconnected from filial discourse or the local community.

This chapter will address the first group, those attempting to tame *jouissance*, while each of the next two will address the resolutions sought by youth in the second and third groups, those of such "substitute" initiations.

The House of Atreus

Viola and Volcaro's (2018) Freudian-Lacanian examination of initiation rites emphasized the importance of ritual pain and scarification in the rites, such that the novice's body is transitioned from an individual's body to a collective body. This is particularly relevant because of the binding of *jouissance* so clearly involved in the process of ritual body modification, not only in giving it form but in structuring the application of it and tying it to identity within the social link. Here again, Lacan's (2011/2018) notion that the body is not necessarily *one* body but a confusion of bodies in which *jouissance* is not localizable except within the bodied field is relevant. *Jouissance* has never been, in the history of speaking beings, something experienced in a solitary fashion. There is always an Other. Without an Other to facilitate the binding of *jouissance*, it remains unbound and troubling.

Thus, ritual scarification and body modification are meant to bind the *jouissance* of youth (Viola & Vorcaro, 2018). Although such binding might be made without the ritual pain or modification characteristic of many cultures in the past (and still a good number in the present), the binding must always—crucially—be embodied. Those youth who are unable to make-do with either traditional or novel initiations are left to cope with an indigestible experience in the body. It is for this reason that supposed "personality features" (a would-be euphemism for "borderline personality disorder" in adolescents) have been increasing in recent years.

Cutting and non-suicidal self-injury (NSSI) more broadly are the most readily apparent examples of makeshift solutions to the problem of initiation. With reference to erotic injury, Lacan (1991/2007) commented that marks upon the skin are "nothing other than a subject identifying itself as the object of *jouissance*" (p. 49). In context, he was referring to marks of flagellation in erotogenic masochism. Freud's (1924) theory of masochism yielded a complex formulation regarding how, exactly, a painful stimulus becomes erotogenic—and it was erotogenic masochism that he believed was at the root of other forms of masochism. Calling upon his *Three Essays on the Theory of Sexuality* (Freud, 1905), he postulated that sexual excitement is always aroused, at least in infantile sexuality, as a secondary consequence of any internal processes exceeding a certain level of quantitative stimulation in the body, including pain and unpleasure, as a sort of "libidinal sympathetic excitation" (Freud, 1924, p. 163). Freud considered that this phenomenon would remain in adulthood depending on "varying degree of development in different sexual constitutions" (p. 163). Nonetheless, this alone was not enough for Freud to explain masochism because of masochism's relationship with sadism. To further elaborate matters, Freud argued that the life drive modifies the death drive such that it would divert some quantity of the death drive to the outside world, not only as direct aggression but in the broader sense of a drive for power over something (*Bemächtigungstrieb*)[1] or the will to power (*Wille zur Macht*). The part directed outward that continues to cling to sexual functioning is "sadism proper," while the part that remains directed inward and clings to sexual functioning is erotogenic masochism (p. 163).

Freud's (1924) notion of the death drives being modified by the life drives and resulting in combinations of masochism and sadism is something he further developed in considering the role of culture (Freud, 1930), although at this later time he argues that the two drives always appear together and makes reference to sadism not as an instance when the life drive modifies the death drive, directing it outward to preserve the individual, but as an instance when the death drive "twists the erotic aim in its own sense" (p. 121).

Notably, Freud's comments in *Civilization and Its Discontents* intimate a more nuanced version of drive theory than a sort of Manichean dualism. Rather than working against each other, the drives always appear in some combined form together, often in ways difficult to ascertain. This provides a clear Freudian foundation for Lacan's later elaborations. In his *Four Fundamental Concepts of Psychoanalysis*, for example, he argued that:

> The distinction between the life drive and the death drive is true in as much as it manifests two aspects of the drive. But this is so only on condition that one sees all the sexual drives as articulated at the level of significations in the unconscious, in as much as what they bring out is death—death as signifier and nothing but signifier...
>
> (Lacan, 1973/1978, p. 257)

This marks a turn away from the pseudo-Manichean reading of Freud's drive theory as a dualism to a quasi-Sabellian modalism, with *the* drive manifesting in one mode or another. This is not necessarily inconsistent with Freud's (1930) position, which held that "libido has a share in every instinctual manifestation [*Triebäußerung*], but that not everything in that manifestation is libido" (p. 121 footnote 1); in other words, despite Freud's view that the energy of the death drive is not libido, libido is nonetheless implicated. Given his previous statement about each drive being intertwined with the other to different degrees in different expressions, it seems a small step to consider this a drive that simply manifests in different ways. Lacan (1973/ 1978) linked signification with the death aspect of the drive, as signification marks the absence of something—as he quoted from St. Paul in the Christian tradition (2 Cor. 3:6), "the letter kills" (Lacan, 1966/2006, p. 719). However, he also related the interconnection of death and sex to the idea of sexed reproduction, which is necessitated by death in contrast to the immortality of asexual reproduction offered at the cellular level. The intertwining of life drives and death drives is a continued development of a position Lacan (1978/1988) took much earlier, in *The Ego in Freud's Theory*, wherein he argued that "the ego is inscribed in the imaginary. Everything pertaining to the ego is inscribed in imaginary tensions, like all the other libidinal tensions. Libido and the ego are on the same side" (p. 326) and that Freud's (1920) *Beyond the Pleasure Principle*:

> is the point where we open out into the symbolic order, which isn't the libidinal order in which the ego is inscribed, along with all the drives. It tends beyond the pleasure principle, beyond the limits of life, and that is why Freud identifies it with the death instinct....The death instinct is only the mask of the symbolic order....
>
> (Lacan, 1978/1988, p. 326)

In this sense, the drive appears in favor of life at the imaginary level and in favor of death at the symbolic level.[2] Lacan's later theorization about the sexual drives being articulated in significations seems less to contradict this earlier position than to modify it—the libido is in a dialectical tension with the signification that articulates it, such that it is alloyed indisputably with death. Interestingly, in Freud's account of masochism in 1924, pleasure and unpleasure are no longer solely quantitative matters—with pleasure involving only the decrease of tension and unpleasure involving the increase of tension. Instead, they also pertain to some mysterious qualitative factor that Freud was unable to define.[3] The imaginary and symbolic registers offer one explanation for such qualitative factors.

The difference between erotogenic masochism and non-erotic self-induced pain or damage is not academic; one can intuitively divine the importance of the difference between stepping into a noose for the purpose of autoerotic asphyxiation and for the purpose of ending one's life. Returning to the notion of NSSI, what distinguishes NSSI from an erotic practice? The sexual excitation in erotic practice is obviously one element, which suggests that what is in both cases an excitation of tension is qualitatively different. Lacan (1991/2007) connected masochism to *jouissance*, with the welt of the whip marking one as the object of *jouissance*. However, in the case of masochism, the question becomes:

> whose *jouissance*? Is it the *jouissance* of whosoever carries what I am calling the glory of the mark? Is it certain that this means the Other's *jouissance*? Certainly, this is one of the ways in which the Other enters one's world, and assuredly, it is an irrefutable one. But the marks' affinity with *jouissance* of the body itself is precisely where it is indicated that it is only through *jouissance*, and *jouissance* alone, that the division distinguishing narcissism from the relation with the object is established.
>
> (p. 49)

Lacan builds here on his ideas regarding perversion (masochism), *jouissance*, and the fantasy. While $S \lozenge a$, the split subject in relation to the object, is the fantasy of the neurotic, the perverse subjective structure is predicated on a different fantasy, one wherein the subject does to accept its position as split but instead never leaves the position of the object of *jouissance* that completes a subject ($a \lozenge S$). In *Formations of the Unconscious*, Lacan (1998/2017) located perverse identification with the object of *jouissance* at the level of a short circuit between the ego and the specular image. In this case, the specular image never has lack introduced into it such that *a* becomes separated from the ego. This is the sense in which the welt marks the subject as the object of *jouissance*, and it is this *jouissance* that reveals the lack of distinction between the ego and the object in perversion. This is an imaginary captation at its core.

In neurosis, however, *jouissance* is not sought but kept at bay by desire. Lacan (1966/2006) stated that "desire is a defense, a defense against going beyond a limit in *jouissance*" (p. 825). In this sense, erotogenic masochism engenders *jouissance* in a libidinal fashion as a qualitatively imaginary experience of a quantitative excitation. In contrast, NSSI is at least in part engaged in with the purpose of delimiting unpleasurable emotional experience (Nock, 2010), placing this form of injury not in the realm of *jouissance* but desire, limiting the excitation of *jouissance*. This is accomplished precisely as Lacan (1973/1978) described in his *Four Fundamental Concepts,* through the functioning of the cut as a signifier. Of course, this is something of a condensation of different positions Lacan took over time; for example, he eventually moved away from the concept of libido and toward *jouissance*, and *jouissance* itself took on a greater association with the death drive. Nevertheless, the use of desire as a defense against *jouissance* is largely consistent with his developments of Freud's theories.

It is in this sense of limiting that self-injury binds *jouissance*. The limitation is both in the form of a localization of *jouissance* in the cut or wound of the body and also in the sense that the excitation is reduced. How such a cut signifies desire, however, requires further consideration of desire's origin in the subject.

The division between the specular image and the object (of the Other's *jouissance*) is the indescribably momentous task of separation, which is effected by the paternal function. This occurs because the subject first sees in the mirror stage an image—the specular image ratified by the parents and which becomes the basis of the ego. It is the relation to this image that first lays the foundation of the fantasy ($S \lozenge a$), a fantasy in which the ego is identified with its imaginary counterpart, the ideal ego or i(a). The ideal ego, the specular image ratified by the parents, is the object, both for the subject and for the Other. The subject assumes its role as this object for the Other in an attempt to prevent the Other from lacking, attempting to prevent from emergence the signifier of lack in the Other, or $S(\cancel{A})$. It is the fact that the Other desires something else—that is, a lack the subject cannot satisfy—that causes a fissure to erupt between i(a) and a. The a falls out of the i(a), becoming the subject's own lost object cause of desire. This is separation—separation of the specular image from the object. What follows is the construction of a tertiary narcissism, that of the ego ideal (I[A]), a symbolic agency that governs the relation to the social link (Moncayo, 2008). In this way, the $S(\cancel{A})$ is the formal cause of neurosis.

I have written previously about the way in which the suppression (*Unterdrückung*) of the $S(\cancel{A})$ leads to a collapse of demand and desire, problems in identification (because of the confusion between the ideal ego and ego ideal), and the great variety of instances of acting out in youth seeking solutions to this problem (Waitz, 2022). In these cases, although the signifier of lack in the Other entered into discourse at the time of subjective structuring, puberty, as Guerra (2020) noted, is a time that calls for more from the Other. When the Other instead seeks to rescind the $S(\cancel{A})$, it is because of a failure of the secondary level of discourse, of the paternal discourse that fails to materialize and cause desire—desire in the sense of both the incompleteness of the maternal discourse within the context of language as well as the incompleteness of the subject with respect to maternal discourse. This semblant of the secondary Other falters. The deployment of acting out by youth serves, in this case, as a way of claiming promissory estoppel, seeking an Other to prevent the Other from going back upon its earlier promise of lack.

At the time, I wrote about suicidal behavior as a form of acting out (Waitz, 2022). In such cases, the mental presentation of the death of the subject serves as a supplement to $S(\cancel{A})$, a way of confronting the Other with an irrevocable lack. Similarly, NSSI becomes a method of reinforcing the paternal function by marking a limit upon the surface of the image. The mark codifies, at the level of the image, a *jouissance* that fills the body, and the mark is visible to the Other as constructed by the subject. The mark, then, is also in part an address in the only register from which the Other appears to receive information (the imaginary). The address forms a question, a version of the *"che vuoi?"* that animates a certain stage of desire's course (Lacan, 1966/2006, p. 690). This is the question Lacan (1991/2007) asked of masochism: Is this my *jouissance* or yours? What must I be to you?

However, the binding of free libido in the localized wound is one version of a larger project of isolating *jouissance* that is not adequately bound within the social link. Another important method of binding *jouissance* can be found in the increasing prevalence of conditions like misophonia or sensory sensitivities, which rely upon the role perception plays as the connecting point between anatomy and psyche (Freud, 1920; 1923; 1939). Perception, in these conditions, serves as a point of entry for what is experienced as an intrusive and foreign *jouissance* without adequate binding within the social link. The sounds typically hated by those who experience misophonia, for example, are those generated by the other—chewing, breathing, coughing, and so on (Vitoratou et al., 2023). The limits established by those with sensory sensitivity (limits such as, although not only, noise canceling headphones, avoidance of family dinners, or punishment of the other in the form of tics) are established to encircle *jouissance* in the sensory input received from the locus of the other, marking a boundary such that if only the input can be dampened, reduced, to stopped, so too can *jouissance*.

One might observe this is a quasi-phobic action, one wherein the purification of the pleasure ego (see Freud, 1915) leads to a displacement of *jouissance* onto the other. This solution is only "quasi" phobic, however, as it does not entail a concomitant projection of aggression; that remains internal. Indeed, irritation is the most common affect associated with the aptly named misophonia (Vitoratou et al., 2023) as the intrusive irruption of the other's *jouissance* into the subject's field of perception is met with an aggressivity aimed to temper such *jouissance*. In NSSI, that aggression is still subjectivized such that it is deployed against the Other. Thus, while Little Hans projected the aggression he felt onto the horse representing his father (Freud, 1909), no projection takes place here.

These similarities notwithstanding, there is a slight difference between the delimitation of *jouissance* in the damage of the imaginary body and in the barriers of perception. The former entails a secondary confusion—a rescission by the Other—of the distinction between the ideal ego and the ego ideal. The latter is a consequence not of such a confusion but of the inability of the social link to socialize *jouissance*. Because the disturbance is between the subject and the other (rather than between two regions of the ego), the regulatory activity is not one by the subject against the body but by the subject against the other as such.

The confusion of the specular image and the object of *jouissance* may occur earlier than in adolescence, although in such a case it would be more accurate to say they are never distinguished rather than that they are confused. Lacanian psychoanalysis broadly categorizes its nosology according to the relationship between the subject and the Other. For those who foreclose the paternal function altogether, refusing any alienation in the social link, the subjective position of psychosis results. This means that, while nonpsychotic subjects have some sense of a distinction between the specular image and the object (some way in which the Other's desire is not entirely encompassed within the subject's image), the person in psychosis has no such separation. They do not experience the alienation of the mirror stage, nor the separation that follows in the installation of the signifier of lack in the Other. Without the i(a)-a division, the psychotic is completely at the mercy of the Other. Because the ego does not fully form, primal repression does not occur, the unconscious is not fully structured, and that which was not repressed returns in the real in the form of hallucinatory experiences (Lacan, 1981/1997).

Lacan followed the tradition of identifying a dichotomy between paranoia and schizophrenia in the psychoses despite similar underlying mechanisms (Redmond, 2013). This dichotomy is less elaborated by introductory secondary texts in English, but is relevant to keep in mind in considering the possibility of numerous configurations of the same underlying structure in Lacanian thought.

In contrast to psychosis, in neurosis, both alienation and separation occur, such that the neurotic is able to incorporate both an ideal ego and an ego ideal. The fantasy of neurosis is what I have referred to as fantasy so far: $ ◊ a. However, neurosis also has two alternate structures within it: the hysteric, whose desire is for an unsatisfied desire, and the obsessional, whose desire is for an impossible desire (Lacan, 1981/1997). Obsession and hysteria are two forms of neurosis in a similar manner that paranoia and schizophrenia are two forms of psychosis. The fantasies in each case animate the psychical operations of neurotics, such that much of one's behavior—whether categorized as an index of illness in descriptive psychiatry or not—may be explicated on their bases.

A separate set of problems arise when alienation occurs and separation does not. In this case, the subject identifies with the object as object of *jouissance*, which is the fantasy of perversion, a ◊ $ (Lacan, 1966/2006). The object in this case completes the Other, disavowing the signifier of lack in the Other (S[Å]). This is connected, of course, to fetishism in the Freudian sense, which is predicated on the disavowal of the mother's castration.

For Lacan, perversion is neither primarily nor always about a sexual fetish but about a relationship to the Other from the position of the object, wherein sadistic relationships are one of completion, the Other being brought to completion either in the body of another subject or in the body of Nature, which licenses the horrors of the Sadean libertine for its own completion/*jouissance*. Generally, the structure of perversion has not been bifurcated by analysis as have psychosis and neurosis.

Nevertheless, some psychoanalysts have attempted to explain the increasing prominence of so-called borderline states by the use of just such a bifurcation. Jean Pierre Lebrun (2012) developed an argument along these lines regarding borderline phenomena, arguing that the subject of the so-called borderline represents a *"perversion ordinaire"* (p. 81), which I paraphrased elsewhere as a distinction "between perversion as a subjective description of one who perverts and perversion as an objective description of the one who is perverted...from [their] course" (Waitz, 2019, p. 35). The subject is, in this formulation, suborned. Lebrun (2012) believed this had to do with the loss of the father, as others have written about, such that it represented a *"mèreversion"* (para. 18) rather than *"pèreversion"* (para. 37). Because of the significance of the maternal in overtaking or suborning the subject, Lebrun oriented these ideas around, rather than an Oedipal scene, and Oresteian one, wherein the subject must pursue the death of the maternal Other in response to the murder of the paternal Other.

To take Lebrun's metaphor a step farther, the house of Atreus is an apt metaphor for U.S. society today. The paternal Other has been called to account again and again in an ever-accelerating series of reckonings that reflect a certain attempt to exact justice from the Other for the sacrifice of Iphigenia on the altar of power—the acts of the paternal Other against the innocent. However, this has resulted in a society without adequate recourse to social structure.

Without the paternal Other's prohibition on *jouissance*, it remains unbound. When the upsurge in real sexual *jouissance* experienced by the subject in puberty places in question once again the desire of the Other, a return to the paternal Other through nomination is necessary. As the Name-of-the-Father, when not foreclosed, metaphorizes the desire of the mother in the Oedipal period, it is this name to which the subject returns, looking again for a seduction, a way of pleasing the Other without being consumed as a matter of *abusus*. The defense against *abusus* is the usufruct Lacan (1975/1998) envisioned, wherein *jouissance* involves the Other's rights of *usus* and *fructus*, but not *abusus*. This is the origin of the term *jouissance*—to enjoy property, according to the three categories of Roman law (Tsujimura & Tsujimura, 2021).

For Lebrun (2012), the subject after the murder of Agamemnon is in the place of Orestes, that is, not one who is gratified by the murder but who plots its recompense through the *lex talionis*. One could argue that this is actually the only true expression of the Electra complex. Lebrun classed this as a form of neurosis, but considered the defense mechanism characteristic of it as a foreclosure of access to the Name-of-the-Father. I have argued previously that such a foreclosure of access seems more consonant with a disavowal rather than a foreclosure, such that *mère-version* would form a pair with *père-version*, bifurcating perversion in a manner similar to psychosis and neurosis (Waitz, 2019). This is the degree to which a change in subjectivity seems to be possible.

Problems of desire are at the center of this psychoanalytic examination of youth mental health. This is because desire is the substrate of subjectivity and it manages the distance of the subject to *jouissance* (Lacan, 1986/1992). The reduction of desire to demand, or the extinction of desire in the rescission of the signifier of lack in the Other, is an existential threat to the subject. In this context, suicide becomes a method of inducing desire in the Other. It is an interpretation of the conditions of existence within the bounds of the Other. It also serves as a nomination of *jouissance* as Other; it marks life as no longer lived for oneself. If suicide, NSSI, and certain sensory symptoms are all solutions to managing *jouissance*, it is because the failure of initiation rites have left a significant gap in the ability of the social link to provide nomination that could bind this real *jouissance* to the imaginary and symbolic identifications that historically have contained *jouissance* through the elaborations of culture (see Guerra, 2020). This is clear in considering that the throughline of the second story of Lacan's (1966/2006) graph of desire begins with *jouissance* on the left and, traveling through S(A̸) and the drive, terminates in castration on the right. Without desire (*d*) traveling the vector that institutes these terms (as in Graph III), the *jouissance* has no path to castration, leaving the subject with a degenerate circuit of desire, a collapsing second stage of the graph that eventuates in either acting out (to reinstate desire) or an immersion in the Other's *jouissance* à la Lebrun's mère-version.

The failure of the paternal discourse to establish desire is aligned with the ascendance of the consumerist discourse. This consumerism—the expectation of satisfied demands—is especially difficult to overcome when the discourse has seeped into the sphere of psychiatry and psychology, which increasingly insist that every diagnosis of descriptive psychiatry is attributable to a variation in anatomical structure or function. The notion of curing mental illness at a biological level, popular in some circles of psychiatric medicine and psychology, is perhaps the most concerning of consumerist ideals, as it implies both that subjectivity can be reduced to the real organism and that deviations from what is considered anatomically normal must be corrected. The consumerist principle here, that there is no need not fully articulable in demand and satisfiable therefore, truly goes on casters with no brakes. When treatment of the psyche becomes medicalized, it subordinates psychiatric treatment to little more than the functions of orthopedics and pedagogy to correct the consumer for not being happy in the correct way. This is why psychotherapeutic treatments are increasingly pedagogical encounters built around the delivery of skills to facilitate the client's ability to utilize their behavior to fully resolve a demand. Freud (1920) himself noted the propensity of those bringing their children to analysis to make assumptions about what is a "cured" child. He described that:

> By a healthy child [parents] mean one who never causes his parents trouble, and gives them nothing but pleasure. The physician may succeed in curing the child, but after that it goes its own way all the more decidedly, and the parents are now far more dissatisfied than before.
>
> (p. 150)

The wish for pleasurable children has become so ingrained in U.S. mental health culture that the National Institute of Mental Health (2021) has promulgated guidance for parents that all "effective" psychotherapies by definition include:

- Teaching the child skills to practice at home or school (between-session "homework assignments").
- Measures of progress (such as rating scales and improvements on "homework assignments") that are tracked over time. (p. 3)

This is, of course, several degrees of fatuous. First, it creates a tautology instead of a distinction between that which is efficacious and that which is effective. Second, it assumes in a superstitious manner that the form taken by many psychotherapies in randomized controlled trials—typically as a manual, with homework, with measurements such as the evaluation of homework—contains the magical properties of efficaciousness rather than simply being the methods of its operationalization and measurement. Third, it dismisses the ample evidence of decades of work regarding psychotherapies not primarily based on skills (see Lilliengren, 2023). Finally, however, it assumes the pedagogical model is fully transposable to psychotherapy. This involves an imposition of tasks upon the child, often by the demand of the parent, in order to produce a cured child.

This is not to suggest that no one benefits from skills-based therapies, but that those who do are receiving what is, in psychoanalytic terms, a treatment by suggestion (Waitz & Bekkeli, 2023). It relies upon the transference to the therapist as the one supposed to know. It is also potentially iatrogenic to the youth for whom these skills are not helpful, leading to treatment demoralization and the belief that they are broken and not able to be fixed.

In addition to these considerations, depression itself is worth consideration as prevalence rates of this diagnosis have increased by 7.7 percent between 2009 and 2019 (Daly, 2022). Depression and malaise have become normalized in youth today, and they have shown trends in recent years that are rather remarkable in a hedonistic society: decreases in sexual activity (Centers for Disease Control and Prevention, 2023), decreases in substance use (Centers for Disease Control and Prevention, 2023), decreases in obtaining driver's licenses (Osaka, 2023), all at the same time as the increases in depression. Of course, these are complex issues that likely do not have only one determinative cause. Nonetheless, these decreases all have in common a refusal of the universal injunction to enjoy. Adolescent rebellion in times past was characterized by the transgression of social norms around enjoyment. This rebellion was, in itself, culturally produced (Viola & Vorcaro, 2018) and arguably a result of the early stages of the consumerist discourse. Why would hedonism promulgate rebellion? In early-stage consumerism, it would prompt greater individual consumption (as more and more consumer demands appear when prohibition becomes less and less vociferous), greater individualization of consumers (who no longer partake of consumption in family units), and orient the subject in all cases towards the consumption of supposedly happiness-inducing products. However, once hedonism has saturated a society, the only rebellion left is the refusal of enjoyment. In late-stage consumerism, when social limitations have eroded sufficiently, the injunction to enjoy takes the subject either to the extreme limits of social approbation or, as if completing full transit through a spherical universe, to the novel rebellion of enjoying non-enjoyment. This is not an enlivening of *jouissance* but a dive into the depths of nihilism, a pleasure that finally causes the confusion Freud (1924) found in masochism—one that appears to be on the side of death. The refusal of the subject to attain happiness despite all the ploys and powers of a consumerist paradise and the latest pharmacological and psychotherapeutic developments is a method of ensuring the sustenance of the subject on the only thing it must have to endure—desire.

In contrast to epidemiological attempts to circumscribe suicidal thoughts and behaviors within the limits of risk factors capable of producing odds ratios (or the machine learning equivalent of this [Bernert et al., 2020]), the theory of initiation rites provides a structural understanding of youth suicidal thoughts and behaviors that is capable of connecting these individual behaviors to the broader societal changes in the US. More than this, the initiation rite theory is also able to organize novel interventions in the social link and guide the singular approach with a given patient that characterizes the Freudian-Lacanian tradition. That psychoanalysis can play such a vital role in the understanding of and response to these severe concerns in such a vulnerable population may go against the zeitgeist of the 21st-century U.S. mental health field; it would be a mistake, however, to count psychoanalysis out as a result of its ill reception among authorities in the field that has become so focused on increasing the ubiquity of manualized models of care. Institutions and authorities of mental health would do well to consider the role that psychoanalysis can play in achieving that which these other treatments cannot (Waitz & Bekkeli, 2023).

Notes

1 Strachey's "instinct for mastery" is somewhat less instructive than it could be in communicating the significance of *Bemächtigungstrieb*. White's (2010) exposition on the matter is helpful in elucidating this, and I borrow here her use of "one possibility" of translation: "a drive to gain power over" (p. 818). White also noted how this marked a long-resisted recognition on Freud's part of something like a drive for power, which is something of a capitulation in his longstanding controversy with Adler (White, 2010).

2 This was Evan's (1996) reading when he was a Lacanian as well.

3 Freud (1924; 1938) theorized this unknown element might be a rhythmic aspect to the experiences of pleasure and unpleasure.

References

Bernert, R. A., Hilberg, A. M., Melia, R., Kim, J. P., Shah, N. H., & Abnousi, F. (2020). Artificial Intelligence and Suicide Prevention: A Systematic Review of Machine Learning Investigations. *International Journal of Environmental Research and Public Health*, 17(16), 5929. doi:10.3390/ijerph17165929.

Centers for Disease Control and Prevention. (2023). *Youth Online*. https://nccd.cdc.gov/Youthonline/App/Default.aspx.

Daly, M. (2022). Prevalence of Depression Among Adolescents in the U.S. From 2009 to 2019: Analysis of Trends by Sex, Race/Ethnicity, and Income. *Journal of Adolescent Health*, 70(3),496. doi:10.1016/j.jadohealth.2021.08.026.

Freud, S. (1905). Three essays on the theory of sexuality. *The Standard Edition of the Complete Psychological Works of Sigmund Freud* (Vol. VII), pp. 123–246. Hogarth Press.

Freud, S. (1909). Analysis of a phobia in a five-year-old boy. *The Standard Edition of the Complete Psychological Works of Sigmund Freud* (Vol. X), pp. 1–150. Hogarth Press.

Freud, S. (1915). Instincts and their vicissitudes. *The Standard Edition of the Complete Psychological Works of Sigmund Freud* (Vol. XIV), pp. 109–140. Hogarth Press.

Freud, S. (1920). Beyond the pleasure principle. *The Standard Edition of the Complete Psychological Works of Sigmund Freud* (Vol. XVIII), pp. 1–64. Hogarth Press.

Freud, S. (1923). The ego and the id. *The Standard Edition of the Complete Psychological Works of Sigmund Freud* (Vol. XIX), pp. 1–66. Hogarth Press.

Freud, S. (1924). The economic problem of masochism. *The Standard Edition of the Complete Psychological Works of Sigmund Freud* (Vol. XIX), pp. 155–170. Hogarth Press.

Freud, S. (1930). Civilization and its discontents. *The Standard Edition of the Complete Psychological Works of Sigmund Freud* (Vol. XXI), pp. 57–146. Hogarth Press.

Freud, S. (1938). An outline of psycho-analysis. *The Standard Edition of the Complete Psychological Works of Sigmund Freud* (Vol. XXIII), pp. 139–208. Hogarth Press.

Freud, S. (1939). Moses and monotheism: Three essays. *The Standard Edition of the Complete Psychological Works of Sigmund Freud* (Vol. XXIII), pp. 1–138. Hogarth Press.

Guerra, A. M. C. (2020). La nominación en la adolescencia. *Affectio Societatis (Medellín)*, 17(33), 112–132. doi:10.17533/udea.affs.v17n33a05.

Lacan, J. (1978). *The four fundamental concepts of psychoanalysis*. J. A. Miller (Ed.). (A. Sheridan, Trans.). W.W. Norton & Co. (Original work published 1973.)

Lacan, J. (1988). *The ego in Freud's theory and in the technique of psychoanalysis*. J. A. Miller (Ed.). (S. Tomaselli, Trans.). W.W. Norton & Co. (Original work published 1978.)

Lacan, J. (1992). *The ethics of psychoanalysis*. J. A. Miller (Ed.). (R. Grigg, Trans.). W. W. Norton & Co. (Original work 1986.)

Lacan, J. (1998). *On feminine sexuality, the limits of love and knowledge*. J. A. Miller (Ed.). (B. Fink, Trans.). W.W. Norton & Co. (Original work published 1975.)

Lacan, J. (2006). *Ecrits*. (B. Fink, Trans.). W.W. Norton & Co. (Original work published 1966.)

Lacan, J. (2007). *The other side of psychoanalysis*. J. A. Miller (Ed.). (R. Grigg, Trans.). W.W. Norton & Co. (Original work published 1991.)

Lacan, J. (2017). *Formations of the Unconscious*. J. A. Miller (Ed.). (R. Grigg, Trans.). Polity. (Original work published 1998.)

Lacan, J. (2018). *...Or worse*. J. A. Miller (Ed.) (A. R. Price, Trans.). Polity. (Original work published 2011.)

Lebrun, P. (2012). Lacan et les états-limites. *Connexions*, 1(97), 77–92.

Lilliengren, P. (2023). A comprehensive overview of randomized controlled trials of psychodynamic psychotherapies. *Psychoanalytic Psychotherapy*, 37(2), 117–140. doi:10.1080/02668734.2023.2197617.

Moncayo, R. (2008). *Evolving Lacanian perspectives for clinical psychoanalysis: On narcissism, sexuation, and the phases of analysis in contemporary culture*. Routledge.

National Institute of Mental Health. (2021). Children and mental health: Is this just a stage? [Grey Literature]. www.nimh.nih.gov/sites/default/files/documents/health/p ublications/children-and-mental-health/children-and-mental-health-is-this-just-a -stage.pdf.

Nock, M. K. (2010). Self-injury. *Annual Review of Clinical Psychology*, 6(1), 339–363. doi:10.1146/annurev.clinpsy.121208.1312580.

Osaka, S. (2023, February 13). "I'll call an Uber or 911": Why Gen Z doesn't want to drive. *The Washington Post*. www.washingtonpost.com/climate-solutions/2023/ 02/13/gen-z-driving-less-uber.

Redmond, J. D. (2013). Contemporary perspectives on Lacanian theories of psychosis. *Frontiers in Psychology*, 4, 350. doi:10.3389/fpsyg.2013.00350.

Tsujimura, K. & Tsujimura, M. (2021). Roman law in the national accounting perspective: Usus, fructus and abusus. *Statistical Journal of the IAOS*, 37(2), 613–628. doi:10.3233/SJI-210810.

Viola, D. T. D. & Vorcaro, A. M. R. (2018). A adolescência em perspectiva: Um exame da variabilidade da passagem à idade adulta entre diferentes sociedades. *Psicologia, Teoria e Pesquisa*, 34. doi:10.1590/0102.3772e3448.

Vitoratou, S., Hayes, C., Uglik-Marucha, N., Pearson, O., Graham, T., & Gregory, J. (2023). Misophonia in the UK: Prevalence and norms from the S-Five in a UK representative sample. *PloS One*, 18(3), e0282777–e0282777. doi:10.1371/journa l.pone.0282777.

Waitz, C. (2019). Immersion in the mother: Lacanian perspectives on borderline states. *The Psychoanalytic Review (1963)*, 106(1), 29–47. doi:10.1521/ prev.2019.106.1.29.

Waitz, C. (2022). Acting out and psychoanalytically informed treatment in inpatient adolescent psychiatry. *Psychoanalytic Psychology*, 39(3), 209–216. doi:10.1037/ pap0000405.

Waitz, C. & Bekkeli, K. (2023). Psychoanalytically informed care and behavioral medicine: Consideration and recommendations for evidence-based practice in institutions. *Psychoanalytic Psychology*. doi:10.1037/pap0000489.

White, K. (2010). Note on "Bemächtigungstrieb" and Strachey's translation as "instinct for mastery". *The International Journal of Psychoanalysis*, 91(4), 811–820. doi:10.1111/j.1745-8315.2010.00354.x.

8 Stigma and Stigmata

St. Francis of Assisi experienced a rare and significant miracle in the Roman Catholic tradition: the appearance of stigmata upon his body. The stigmata are the five marks of Christ's wounds at the crucifixion—marks upon the hands and feet as well as the side (Muessig, 2020). The stigmata have a lengthy history in Catholicism, often considered as beginning with St. Francis in 1224 CE and continuing to the present.

The stigmata traditionally appear to those who have the proper disposition, developed in the process of growing in Christlikeness, especially as it relates Christ's passion (Muessig, 2020). Muessig noted that one 19th-century historian of stigmata considered "the stigmatic as a person in deep contemplation of the Man of Sorrows, thereby engulfed in a 'sea of wretchedness' and compassionate suffering" (p. 5). Notably, the stigmata are associated with both pain and a transcendental enjoyment, sometimes with a sense of a piercing of the heart, not unlike the transverberation of St. Theresa of which Lacan (1975/1998) made much in the 20th year of his published seminar. The stigmata are animated by a *jouissance* bound in the marks through a nomination as Christlike. The nomination delivered by the marks thus plays the role of binding the real of *jouissance*, the imaginary body, and the symbolic ego ideal together for the subject. This sort of binding of real, imaginary, and symbolic became increasingly important to Lacan later in his career. In the 23rd year of his seminar, he elaborated the three registers (real, imaginary, symbolic) as cords bound in a Borromean link (Lacan, 2005/2016). However, this link can fail, leading to psychic disquietude. In considering this, Lacan introduced his conception of the *sinthome*, a fourth cord that binds the other three together. The *sinthome*, an older spelling of *symptôme* in French, is a creation of the subject with which the subject identifies, a way of deploying the symptom that is workable for the subject through a real identification.

Verhaeghe and Declercq (2002) describe the *sinthome* as a real suppletion of the failing of the Name of the Father. In neurosis proper, the Name of the Father does not require suppletion as it acts as a metaphor for the lack in the Other, taking the position of S(Ⱥ). However, when this fails, suppletion is required. Symbolic suppletion is an alternative to real suppletion, and

DOI: 10.4324/9781032666334-12

Verhaeghe and Declercq argue that "the belief in the symptom is the Symbolic suppletion for the lack of the Other" (p. 69). The belief in the symptom is a belief that the symptom requires the delivery of a final meaning in order to unravel the suffering associated with the symptom; this is contrasted with identification with the symptom in the *sinthome*. Thus, one's relationship to the symptom might be belief in or identification with. Such belief in the symptom characterizes especially the early stage of analysis, when the analysand presents to the analyst with the transference of supposing they know what the symptom means. However, at a certain moment in the treatment, the analysand is faced with the dichotomous choice: "either he chooses a new solution and identifies with the Real of the symptom; or he sticks to the previous solution and looks for yet another meaning by way of another hysterical identification: $\math600 \rightarrow S1 \rightarrow S2$" (p. 68).

However, Vanheule (2016) argued that subjects in the age of the capitalist discourse no longer reliably attribute a meaning to their symptom, such that transference is not necessarily expected any longer in the psychoanalytic setting. This complicates the notion of a belief in the symptom, as such a belief is no longer in the symbolic content of the symptom but in the imaginary status of the symptom as a biological malfunction. I noted elsewhere that transference in this context is a transference to the one supposed to know about the malfunction of the body and its supposedly behavioral sequelae (Waitz & Bekkeli, 2023), to which I might add that the one who knows in many such cases is expected to validate the permanence of the symptom rather than to implement its cure. Vanheule (2016) characterized the theorization of analysts around the new development of subjectivity in capitalist discourse as a move from "conflict and impossibility in relation to the other" to "crises in response to a confrontation with the fundamental non-rapport" (p. 9). This seems consonant with the shift from the centering of lack to the centering of loss.

Notably, Lacan (2005/2016) played on the homophony of *sinthome* with other terms, such as *saint homme*, the holy man. As Vanheule (2016) noted, this reflects Lacan's view of one's *savoir faire*, a knowing what to do with one's symptom. The saint, as in St. Francis, exhibits a knowing what to do with in the institution of the stigmata. Importantly, the language of stigmata is that of marking rather than wounding. If the latter were at issue, one might speak of traumata. That it is a stigma rather than a trauma is indicative of the way in which lack rather than loss is at stake. Stigma also has a conceptual history in ancient Greek culture, wherein the stigma was the practice of marking or tattooing the bodies of those in society who ought to be shunned (Tyler, 2020). Thus, more than a wound, the ancient stigmata assigned a place in social discourse to the recipient, even if one of abjection. By marking those who have deviated from the societally approved trajectory, the ancient stigmatized found themselves both included within (by being accounted for) and excluded from (by being marginalized) the social order. In a certain sense, like their Catholic cognates, the ancient stigmata also bind *jouissance* through a naming, a naming of the transgressive *jouissance* of the bearer.

To collect these ideas of stigma, stigmata, stigmatization, and stigmatics is more than interesting wordplay. Their juxtaposition allows for some interesting observations. A first observation in this juxtaposition is that psychoanalysis can shed the light of ambivalence upon stigma, problematizing the one-sided interpretation of stigma as uniformly damaging at the social level. This creates play for more nuanced and intricate understanding of stigma.

Second, and relatedly, there is a tension between the abjection of the stigmatized and the ecstasy of the stigmatic. This tension is also encapsulated by Lacan's (1974/1990) slightly different take on sainthood in *Television*: that the analyst is a saint. However, a saint here is not one who practices *caritas* but "*trashitas*" (p. 15). That is, "the saint is the refuse of *jouissance*" (p. 16). In this sense, the saint is indifferent to *jouissance*, allowing the subject (analysand) to become "aware of his position, at least within the structure" (p. 15). The saint, then, is mortified to *jouissance* but not without use for the subject as an object of desire.

The precise duality located at the node of stigma and stigmata—both acting as a method of binding *jouissance* and attended by the ambivalence of being set apart—is the unity of the sacred, wherein that which is set apart is fully invested with transcendent truth and located in the categories of both holy and profane. This is akin to the *homo sacer* figure of Roman law.[1]

A similar concept is that of the mechanism of scapegoating. Beyond its casual, metaphorical use in proverbial English, the scapegoat has its origins in the ancient Hebrew tradition of investing a goat, through ritual practice, with the sin of the people (Lev. 16). This was the goat was dedicated to Azazel, although whether this speaks to sending the goat into the desert or as a dedication to an evil spirit is ambiguous (Finlan, 2005). Freud's (1915) explication of the purification of the pleasure ego is satisfactory in itself as an understanding of scapegoating, wherein the objectionable content of the ego is displaced onto the external object of the goat.

The scapegoating process is closely related to the unipolar reading of stigmatization, that the normality of the people is predicated on the exclusion of a subset of others from the social link. This is the common reading of stigmatization, as a review of public health literature will reflect. Nevertheless, this is the space wherein psychoanalysis might serve to problematize settled understandings at the level of colloquial truisms.

If the role of stigmatization as a negative social determinant of health is one side, what is the other side of stigmata? This is a challenging question that should not be considered lightly. It is similar in many ways to the evolution of Freud's (1897) "*neurotica*" (p. 264), his seduction theory in which he initially argued that neuroses proceeded from child sexual abuse. In the face of what he viewed as the improbability of facts surrounding his theory, Freud began to consider the importance of sexual fantasy in the life of children given the ambiguity in the unconscious between fantasy and reality, leading to Freud's (1914) conclusion that "this psychical reality requires to be taken into account alongside practical reality" (pp. 17–18). It should be noted, however, that this never led Freud to discount the reality of child sexual abuse, as he maintained that such events are relatively common (Freud, 1938). Thus, the widening of psychoanalytic understanding to include psychic reality is not exclusive to the consideration of historical fact; however, it does shift the focus of psychoanalysis from the strictly factual to the fantasy, or fantasm, that structures the subject. The construction of the fantasm is always an active engagement by the subject of the unconscious, rendering even the most extreme of circumstances open to differential impact on the basis of the fantasm's filtering of sensory perception. This is why Lacan (1973/1978) emphasized the fundamental activity of the drive, moving from the active, reflexive, passive series to a statement marking the activity of the drive even in supposedly passive phases: "*making oneself seen*" instead of being seen, for example (p. 200). The subject is always active.

The activity of the drive in constructing the fantasy is of central importance in considering the other side of stigmatization. Not everyone who experiences stigmatization undergoes the same process. For some, stigmatization is incidental to subjectivity while for others, it is central. In a sense, this is the distinction between stigma as a mark and stigmata as a transcendental efflorescence of *jouissance*, which comes to the surface. Stigmata act, as perhaps they did for St. Francis, as a form of suppletion of the Name of the Father, but is it symbolic or real in Verhaeghe and Declercq's (2002) sense? Is this an identification with, or a belief in, the symptom?

To add some flesh to this discussion, one might consider the mass psychogenic illnesses of the early 2020s. A prime example of this is the explosion of functional tic and Tourette disorders among youth—especially girls—in the early period of the COVID-19 pandemic pursuant to increasing exposure to information and misinformation about these disorders on social media (Frey et al., 2022). This marked a significant outbreak of psychogenic symptom via the internet in contrast to earlier forms of mass psychogenic illness requiring physical proximity (Hull & Parnes, 2021). The reason for the spread of functional tic and Tourette symptoms in youth is open to debate, although isolation in the pandemic and increased stress are typically cited along with increases in depression and anxiety (Frey et al., 2022), but these do not explain the specificity of tic and Tourette symptoms. For example, why would isolation not simply increase depression and anxiety? In what way would it contribute to functional tic or Tourette symptoms on top of this? What would the mechanism be of depression and anxiety as contributors to these functional symptoms? Organic and physiological substrates of functional movement disorders have also been investigated (Drane et al., 2021), although this does not necessarily address, for example, the ability of functional symptoms to be communicated via digital exposure or why so many more youth would exhibit these functional symptoms in such a unique moment of history (unless one argues that there is a large number of people with "untriggered" physiological conditions ripe for psychogenic illness that, for some reason, have not occurred otherwise).

Despite the contemporary derogation of Freudian psychoanalysis within the broader mental health field, it is remarkable that the ideas Freud outlined regarding social contagion in 1921 have continuing relevance. Freud elaborated social contagion as a form of "identification based upon the possibility or desire of putting oneself in the same situation" as another seen exhibiting a symptom (p. 107). This is the form of identification Freud explicitly noted required no relationship with the object of identification. However, the fact that this is a form of identification does not resolve the question of *identification with* or *belief in* from the perspective of Verhaeghe and Declercq (2002), who argued that these are, in fact, "two radically different forms of identification" (p. 67). In light of Freud's (1921) theorization, the explanation of causality of social contagion must be investigated from the perspective of what, in social media representations of the mark (stigma) of illness, youth have seen and desired for themselves.

Recognizing that the failure of initiation rites has created an environment in the US of a decreasingly potent Name of the Father, the suppletion of the Name of the Father is of increasing psychic importance. If youth are accomplishing such suppletion through the adoption of functional symptoms, how does this operate? The disintegration of larger orders of meaning has precipitated disintegration in Durkheim's (1897/1997) sense, leaving youth without a sense of community or identity that credibly supports subjectivity. There are three especially intriguing aspects to this with respect to the adoption by youth of stigmatized symptom-identities.

First, I have heard numerous youth discuss the way in which having a particular diagnosis would induct them into a larger community. For example, youth seeking the diagnosis of dissociative identity disorder without meeting criteria for such might discuss the importance they have found in online communities celebrating being plural or being a system. This sense of integration within an online community is highly appealing—as one would expect of any highly cohesive community—and motivating for receiving a diagnosis. This is not to say that such youth do not experience something in their psyche that connects them to a specific community; however such community is often of primary interest to youth who are alienated in society more broadly, lacking any meaningful induction.

Second, and similarly, many youth discuss the importance of a diagnosis for meaning making. Their language often suggests that if they receive a certain diagnosis, it will *explain* much of their experience or their childhood. For example, with respect to the increasing number of socially typical youth seeking diagnoses of autism, it is noteworthy that the typical grounds for seeking this diagnosis are (1) to explain the subjective sense of peculiarity; and (2) to justify a subjective sense of engagement in socially inappropriate behaviors. In both instances, the failure of initiation rites to integrate youth into society appears implicated. The liminal rite of initiation extends indefinitely in such cases, and, without a rite of incorporation and the nomination promulgated therein that governs belongingness in the social link, a sense of alienation in the social link becomes fixed. A new identification must be located that creates within a new social bond a meaning for the alienation experienced in the rite of separation; the novice essentially must stitch together two different rites of initiation, with incorporation into a new link constructing a retroactive understanding of the first two rites involved in separating from the old link.

Regarding socially inappropriate behaviors, the nomination of autism provides a (putatively) neurological justification for such behaviors of the subject. Aggressivity (making hurtful comments, ignoring social cues, and so on) is thus displaced from the subject who is no longer implicated once neurology is implicated. The logic becomes *I am off-putting to others not because of my subjective position towards them but because I am autistic.* One example of this is a patient, whom a reputable neuropsychologist determined did not have autism but something closer to conversion or factitious disorder related to autism, coming to treatment repeatedly stating a demand to learn more socially acceptable behaviors (acceptable to peers and to family) yet staunchly opposed to any movement toward change in this direction, whether through direct suggestion or the gentlest of open-ended inquiries. This patient was aware of social cues by their own discussion of having not responded to them. They would intentionally ignore opportunities for engaging in socially acceptable behaviors with their friends due to not wanting to "mask" their symptoms, and they would similarly scream at their parents when the parents did not do as they wished. In cases like this, the role of the diagnosis sought is both to integrate one into one form of social link but also to reify the exclusion from society at the level of biology. When one considers the psychic weight of disintegration in Durkheim's (1897/1997) sense, it seems reasonable for youth to seek ways to explain and justify this alienation and—why not?—the anger underlying their sense of exclusion. When the social link has failed, it is no wonder that youth, finding themselves outside the social link and uncertain how to enter it, look for a nomination that could bind the *jouissance* related to this experience in a new way.

This is also related to the third aspect of youth adopting stigmatized identities, namely, the embodiment of being an outlaw (*homo sacer*), one for whom the law does not apply. Because one has not been integrated into society, there is an almost juridical push in some cases to confront the Other with that which it has refused, as if to say "since you do not want me as part of you, you must put up with the fact that your rules do not apply to me." This is most evident in the functional coprolalia that is different from its more traditional Tourette or tic counterparts in part due to the coprolalia in functional cases containing longer strings of complex phrases, a wider array of inappropriate words employed, and statements occurring in pauses and in a different pitch than ongoing conversation (Ganos et al., 2016). Such occurrences can be viewed easily on any number of social media accounts with millions of followers. They can also be heard in the stories of patients reporting tic disorders in which they, for example, tell a peer to "shut up" involuntarily when the peer is annoying or in cursing in someone's presence when they are angry with them. However, this confrontation with the Other is also similar to those interactions described in the previous chapter, wherein a quasi-phobic provocation of the Other requires the Other's presentification to the subject such that it confirms its existence.

The return of the socially excluded in the form of involuntary behaviors reflects a transformation of stigma to stigmata, a form of confronting the Other in a particular fashion that requires a centering of subjectivity on the involuntary acts apparently necessitated by the Other (in the form of Nature, or the reified physiological underpinnings that are permanent and irrevocable). With this in mind, one might return to the question of the choice described by Verhaeghe and Declercq (2002) between two forms of identification: *identification with* the symptom as in the *sinthome* or *belief in* the symptom as in the continual *dérobade* of hysteria. The adoption of the *sinthome*, the acceptance of responsibility of *jouissance* such as one finds in the story of St. Teresa of Avila, is not the primary role of such functional symptoms. Instead, one finds a position that paradoxically reinforces the Other in the position of the master. This is because there is both a way in which the youth finds a place within the Other's social order through a label—a diagnosis within a credible taxonomy constructed by those who know—as well as a way in which the youth places *jouissance* on the side of the Other (of Nature) who compels the youth's behavior. In this way, the Name of the Father as both integration and regulation is brought to suppletion by the youth.

It is in this sense that one can speak of stigmata when discussing the stigma of a mental health diagnosis. The stigmata represent not an Other *jouissance* but a *jouissance* of the Other bound in certain suffering that is able at the symbolic level of meaning to bind some degree of *jouissance* in an identification with an ego ideal.

Thus, some portion of the crisis of youth mental health is a result of youth seeking incorporation through a symbolic nomination to which they have access, a symptom, as more and more youth seek fashionable diagnoses, including youth who do not reflect the descriptive nosology of the condition as such. This puts the clinician—psychoanalytic or not—in a precarious position. Should the clinician deliver a diagnosis for the salutary effects its reception might have, regardless of its accuracy, the clinician is little more than a functionary who affirms the ideals of the ego—the ego ideal by offering symbolic nomination and the ideal ego by affirming the identity between the ideal ego and the specular image—*you are exactly who you think you are.* Should the clinician deny the diagnosis in a definitive manner, however, this neither moves the youth toward a position of assuming subjective responsibility nor enhances their material wellbeing in the sense of the pleasure ego.

The difficult position of the clinician is that of holding a space for that which is neither one thing nor the other—neither taking the side of the specular image nor falling into the pit of the *dérobade*, as this false exclusive disjunction is a trap. Although some subset of youth will withdraw from treatment when the clinician declines to accede to the position of satisfying their demands for a diagnosis, those who are able to remain and curiously explore their position with respect to their symptom will be able to carry out psychoanalytic work.

Annie Rogers (2017) describes this process, "the analyst's act of making space for naming the unrepresented," as playing the role of the Father of the Name (p. 199). This expression, Father of the Name, is an inversion Lacan (2005/2016) made of his own earlier formulation of the Name of the Father. The Name of the Father executes separation and mediates the passage of the child from the family into society, where, traditionally, the father's name governs the distinction of one family from another—a distinction only needed once one leaves the immediate family, wherein one name (the given name) is enough for distinction. However, the Name of the Father is not quite enough. Guerra (2020) described how, while the Name of the Father operated once as a guarantee or foundation of the symbolic—the Other of the Other—the Name of the Father has since slipped, becoming depredated or, in Guerra's view, foreclosed in culture. This foreclosure in culture, although not leading to mass psychosis because of continued operation at the Oedipal level, leaves pubertal novices in a tenuous position with respect to the binding of the real, imaginary, and symbolic. The Name of the Father is no longer a semblance. These three rings, which Lacan (2005/2016) elaborated in terms of topology, become frayed as discussed above, such that a new intervention is required. For Guerra (2020), this is a separate execution from the Name of the Father in the Oedipal period and is, instead, about the Father of the Name.

The Father of the Name is the function that executes nomination in the form of a tying together of the real, imaginary, and symbolic, even when these are bound by a false knot (Lacan, 2005/2016). Notably, the Father of the Name and the Name of the Father are closely related; Lacan said that "the Name of the Father is also the Father of the Name" (p. 13) and, at another moment, that "the father…as he who names" is "the fourth element" in addition to the real, symbolic, and imaginary (p. 147). Moreover, this fourth element is what Lacan used to "crown what is involved in the Name of the Father" and said it is "what it would be most suitable to call *the sinthome*" (p. 147). If there is a certain consistency between the *sinthome* and the Father of the Name, it is in that the Father of the Name delivers the nomination that could be a *sinthome*, could bind the orders of the psyche together. The relationship between the Father of the Name and the Name of the Father is more complex, however.

Guerra (2020) distinguishes the Name of the Father as erstwhile semblance from the Father of the Name as a function producing a multiplicity of names. For Lacan in his later years, the Father ultimately has not one name but names, which he indicated as early as 1963, when he titled the seminar he refused to complete after his removal as a training analyst of the *Société Française de Psychanalyse* "The Names of the Father" (Lacan, 2005/2013). He continued to refer to this seminar throughout the years, alluding to its contents while never fully elaborating them, treating the seminar like a MacGuffin. Among such comments, Lacan (1974) noted that one Name of the Father is "this one of the masked Man" (p. 33). Not only this:

> but the Father has so many, many [masks] that there is not One that suits him, except the Name of the Name of the Name. No-Name is his Proper Name except for the Name as ex-sistence.
>
> (p. 34)

The Father, then, who fails as a semblance is a series of masks that mask the void Lacan continually placed at the center of the psyche, the sexual non-rapport that "makes a hole in the real" (p. 33). It is this hole that is veiled by the series of masks of the Father, which is another way of saying the Father's many names. Guerra (2020) noted that the pubertal novice must invent a new name, one that goes beyond the Name of the Father's symbolic role and instead provide some form of semblance such that the real, imaginary, and symbolic hang together. Williams (2017) elaborated Lacan's development of the Father through the ultimate equivalence between the Father and the symptom, or *sinthome*, wherein "the Real of the paternal function is to name an instance of *jouissance* such that its jumping up is localised to the same place," thereby "introduc[ing] the function of the symptom" (p. 194).

The *jouissance* of puberty places stress on the semblance of the father that no longer holds together in most of U.S. society. The pubertal novice today must search for some Father of the Name capable of providing a nomination that allows a binding of the real, imaginary, and symbolic. For Lacan (2005/2016), the *sinthome* is "what is singular to each individual" (p. 147) and is ultimately a necessity of the speaking being, such that "there can be no radical reduction of the fourth term [*sinthome*], not even in analysis" (p. 30). This suggests, to the extent that the symptom of nomination through diagnosis is at times mutable, every symptom is not necessarily a *sinthome*. Indeed, one remarkable feature of many instances of nomination for youth today is that they must be stacked. Youth will then share a series of complex intersectional identities, finding a chain of names that incorporate gender, race, diagnosis, disability, and so on, as though placing them in a collection could finally create the semblance that has dissipated around the Father.

Nevertheless, the stigmata of the symptom allows a functioning of the pleasure ego through integration into a community that is set apart in a way ambiguous, such that there is both a curse of discrimination as well as a blessing (*blessure*, perhaps) of pride. This search for some definitive nomination animates one portion of the apparent youth mental health crisis, with diagnoses accumulating in order to govern one's entrance into the social bond. While it is not the role of the psychoanalyst to "correct" errors in descriptive psychiatry, it does fall upon the psychoanalyst to hold the space needed to find a pathway from the symptom to the *sinthome*, such that the youth involved may take up a role of responsibility within their own experience rather than continue in their suffering to be subject to the whims of the Other.

Note

1 This is not an explicit reference to Agamben, but his work has popularized this concept. See Dauber (2024).

References

Dauber, N. (2023). The sacred in the civil law: the Homo Sacer and Sacratae Leges of the legal humanists. *History of European Ideas*, 50(1), 125–152. doi:10.1080/01916599.2023.2233334.

Drane, D. L., Fani, N., Hallett, M., Khalsa, S. S., Perez, D. L., & Roberts, N. A. (2021). A framework for understanding the pathophysiology of functional neurological disorder. *CNS Spectrums*, 26(6), 555–561. doi:10.1017/S1092852920001789.

Durkheim, E. (1997). *Suicide*. G. Simpson (Ed.). (J. A. Spaulding & G. Simpson, Trans.). Free Press. (Original work published 1897.)

Finlan, S. (2005). *Problems with atonement*. Liturgical Press.

Freud, S. (1897). Letter from Freud to Fliess, September 21, 1897. *The Complete Letters of Sigmund Freud to Wilhelm Fliess, 1887–1904* (Vol. XLII), pp. 264–267. Belknap Press.

Freud, S. (1914). On the history of the psycho-analytic movement. *The Standard Edition of the Complete Psychological Works of Sigmund Freud* (Vol. XIV), pp. 1–66. Hogarth Press.

Freud, S. (1915). Instincts and their vicissitudes. *The Standard Edition of the Complete Psychological Works of Sigmund Freud* (Vol. XIV), pp. 109–140. Hogarth Press.

Freud, S. (1921). Group psychology and the analysis of the ego. *The Standard Edition of the Complete Psychological Works of Sigmund Freud* (Vol. XVIII), pp. 65–144. Hogarth Press.

Freud, S. (1938). An outline of psycho-analysis. *The Standard Edition of the Complete Psychological Works of Sigmund Freud*, (Vol. XXIII), pp. 139–208. Hogarth Press.

Frey, J., Black, K. J., & Malaty, I. A. (2022). TikTok Tourette's: Are we witnessing a rise in functional tic-like behavior driven by adolescent social media use? *Psychology Research and Behavior Management*, 15, 3575–3585. doi:10.2147/PRBM.S359977.

Ganos, C., Edwards, M. J., & Müller-Vahl, K. (2016). "I swear it is Tourette's!": On functional coprolalia and other tic-like vocalizations. *Psychiatry Research*, 246, 821–826. doi:10.1016/j.psychres.2016.10.021.

Guerra, A. M. C. (2020). La nominación en la adolescencia. *Affectio Societatis (Medellín)*, 17(33), 112–132. doi:10.17533/udea.affs.v17n33a05.

Hull, M. & Parnes, M. (2021). Tics and TikTok: Functional Tics Spread Through Social Media. *Movement Disorders Clinical Practice (Hoboken, N.J.)*, 8(8), 1248–1252. doi:10.1002/mdc3.13267.

Lacan, J. (1974). Preface to Spring Awakening. Retrieved from https://lacanianworksex change.net/wp-content/uploads/2023/07/19740901SpringAwakeningLacan.pdf.

Lacan, J. (1978). *The four fundamental concepts of psychoanalysis*. J. A. Miller (Ed.). (A. Sheridan, Trans.). W.W. Norton & Co. (Original work published 1973.)

Lacan, J. (1998). *On feminine sexuality, the limits of love and knowledge*. J. A. Miller (Ed.). (B. Fink, Trans.). W.W. Norton & Co. (Original work published 1975.)

Lacan, J. (2013). *On the names of the father*. J. A. Miller (Ed.). (B. Fink, Trans.). Polity. (Original work published 2005.)

Lacan, J. (2016). *The sinthome*. J. A. Miller (Ed.). (A. R. Price, Trans.). Polity. (Original work published 2005.)

Muessig, C. (2020). *The stigmata in medieval and early modern Europe*. Oxford University Press.

Rogers, A. (2017). The Father of the Name: A child's analysis through the last teachings of Lacan. In C. Owens & S. Farrelly Quinn (Eds), *Lacanian psychoanalysis with babies, children, and adolescents: Further notes on the child*, pp. 199–214. Routledge.

Tyler, I. (2020). *Stigma: The machinery of inequality*. Zed Books.

Vanheule, S. (2016). Capitalist discourse, subjectivity and Lacanian Psychoanalysis. *Frontiers in psychology*, 7, 1948. doi:10.3389/fpsyg.2016.01948.

Verhaeghe, P. & Declercq, F. (2002). Lacan's analytical goal: "Le Sinthome" or the feminine way. In L. Thurston (Ed.), *Essays on the final Lacan: Re-inventing the symptom*, pp. 59–83. The Other Press.

Waitz, C. & Bekkeli, K. (2023). Psychoanalytically informed care and behavioral medicine: Consideration and recommendations for evidence-based practice in institutions. *Psychoanalytic Psychology*. doi:10.1037/pap0000489.

Williams, M. (2017). To invent a father…. In C. Owens & S. Farrelly Quinn (Eds), *Lacanian psychoanalysis with babies, children, and adolescents: Further notes on the child*, pp. 185–194. Routledge.

9   The Loss of Not Knowing

Ambivalence, ambiguity, the hermeneutic of suspicion, and the subject's role in its own suffering—these psychoanalytic pillars are increasingly incompatible with social discourse in the United States (including within psychoanalytic groups) which has become more and more polarized in an escalating series of dogmatic certainties. The polarization of the political environment in the United States has become endemic, so much so that social sorting has led members of both primary political parties further away from any ideological overlap or moderation in the middle (Desilver, 2022). Ambiguity is not a selling point for a politician.

This polarization has many causes and contributors. For example, the nonpartisan Carnegie Endowment for International Peace identified three formal factors that make the US especially vulnerable to polarization (McCoy & Press, 2022). The first such factor is the first-past-the-post electoral system. Duverger (1972) long ago described the way in which winner-take-all majority votes on a single ballot inherently privilege a two-party system that over-represents some groups (the winning party) while under-representing others. This system leads smaller voting groups or parties to consolidate resources into larger blocs in order to win elections, ultimately consolidating into two meaningful parties. The US is one of only "three established democracies us[ing] exclusively first-past-the-post plurality voting to choose their legislators" (McCoy & Press, 2022, p. 9). This results in binary decision making that incentivizes partisan sorting in order to increase the share of voters captured in a party's constituency. This is compounded by the other unique structural elements of the U.S. political system, such as strong protections for the minority party, non-proportionate representation in the Senate, and the Electoral College, all of which contribute to gridlock and outcomes that, while mechanically correct, do not represent the electorate proportionately.

A second vulnerability in the US for polarization is the way in which this binary party system encourages parties to exploit further binary logic to mix together social and political identities, a system "in which the two parties reinforce urban-rural, religious-secular, and racial-ethnic cleavages rather than promote cross-cutting cleavages" (McCoy & Press, 2022, p. 7). The tie

DOI: 10.4324/9781032666334-13

between social and political identities contributes to affective polarization, and researchers with the National Bureau of Economic Research noted the connection in research literature between "mass polarization" and "the extent to which a person's political party is aligned with other aspects of the person's identity, such as their race or religion" (Boxell et al., 2021, p. 11). In other words, the first-past-the-post system supports a binary sorting of the electorate, which in turn motivates the two political parties to rely on binary social identities to capture greater shares of voters, leading to social sorting that increasingly alloys social and political identities that charge polarization with a strong affective component.

The Carnegie Endowment for International Peace observed a third vulnerability in the US to polarization: identity politics (McCoy & Press, 2022). While other large multiracial and multicultural democracies exist, McCoy and Press believed the US might be alone in the demographic shift it is undergoing and which may contribute to tensions between demographic groups across lines of race and ethnicity. This may be true, but other large, diverse democracies—such as Brazil and India—are running into similar problems of polarization (Sahoo, 2020; Stuenkel, 2021) regardless of whether a demographic shift is occurring. Nonetheless, the emphasis of political parties on image-based identities has contributed, as discussed in Chapter 4, to the disintegration of a common social identity. These image-based—or imaginary, in Lacanian terms—identities inherently exclude the lack that characterizes the symbolic; the image contains all. As a result, the fifth discourse, predicated as it is on the suppression of lack, has come to dominate the structure of politics in the US in addition to the economy, reaching an apex of illimitable dominion irrespective of political content filling the form (i.e., affecting both the right and left). Consumerism has permeated politics, with "retail politics" and ad purchases gaining as much or more news coverage as policy positions. The image projected by politicians has become even more important than the substance of their character. Overall, the affective polarization impacting the US has increased tolerance across the board for political violence and undemocratic actions of political leaders (McCoy & Press, 2022). Members of the other party are perceived as an existential threat.

These vulnerabilities within the US at the level of political structure have been exploited not only domestically by political parties but by foreign adversaries as well. Aleksandr Dugin, for example, is a far-right Russian ideologue whose work has influenced Russian nationalism, so much so that he was subject to an assassination attempt after the onset of the Russian war in Ukraine (Roth & Farrer, 2022). One of his most important works, *Foundations of Geopolitics*, contained broad visions for a resurgent Russian empire (Dugin, 1997). In this work, Dugin explicitly called for "introduc [ing] geopolitical disorder into internal American activity, encouraging all kinds of separatism and ethnic, social and racial conflicts, actively supporting all dissident movements—extremist, racist, and sectarian groups, thus destabilizing internal political processes in the US" (as cited in Dunlop, 2004, para. 43). He specifically argued for targeting African Americans as a way to inflame backlash against the US. The U.S. Senate's Select Committee on Intelligence reported Russian use of disinformation and social media was deployed in a manner consistent with Dugin's vision during the 2016 U.S. presidential election (S. Rep. No. 116-XX, 2019). Specifically:

> The Committee found that no single group of Americans was targeted by IRA [Internet Research Agency; Russian actors] information operatives more than African-Americans. By far, race and related issues were the preferred target of the information warfare campaign designed to divide the country in 2016. Evidence of the IRA's overwhelming operational emphasis on race is evident in the IRA's Facebook advertisement content (over 66 percent contained a term related to race) and targeting (locational targeting was principally aimed at "African-Americans in key metropolitan areas with well-established black communities and flash-points in the Black Lives Matter movement"), its Facebook pages (one of the IRA's top performing pages, "Blacktivist," generated 11.2 million engagements with Facebook users), its Instagram content (five of the top 10 Instagram accounts were focused on African-American issues and audiences), its Twitter content (heavily focused on hot button issues with racial undertones, such as the NFL kneeling protests), and its YouTube activity (96 percent of the IRA's YouTube content was targeted at racial issues and police brutality).
>
> (pp. 38–39)

However, Russian disinformation targeted Americans across demographic groups and political lines, alternatively pushing conservatives towards voting for Trump and others toward voting for candidates other than Clinton or boycotting the election.

This is the social context—predicated on the image, without room for difference, and intentionally constructed to heighten polarization—in which youth are coming of age, without the guidance of a rite of initiation. That the current rising generation, "Gen Z," is more politically active than its antecedents might reflect a way in which such political engagement can serve as a rite of incorporation (Medina, 2023). It is also true that the rising generation is more liberal than older cohorts (Parker et al., 2019), which may hold true despite the truism of voters growing conservative as they age. For example, more than twice as many Gen Z identify as Democrat versus Republican, revealing a significant polarization gap within the generation (Chinni & Stamm, 2023).

While this may seem peripheral to the youth mental health crisis, some data suggest there is actually an important connection. Gimbrone et al. (2022) found that the mental health of liberal youth began diverging from their conservative peers around the year 2012 (although conservative youth mental health began to worsen shortly after this, around 2013 [for males] and 2014 [for females]). Gimbrone et al. attempt to explain the disparity between political dispositions by appealing to external reality for worsening liberal youth mental health—climate change, school shootings, sexism—and to internal factors protecting conservative youth mental health, stating that "conservative ideology may work as a psychological buffer by harmonizing an idealized worldview with the bleak external realities experienced by many" (p. 7). This is a rather blithe leap from the data to opinion without regard for competing hypotheses. Michelle Goldberg (2023) pointed out the poor fit of this hypothesis with the data, noting that the uptick in liberal mental illness did not follow from Trump's 2016 election but from a largely liberal social milieu in 2012. Instead, she argued that "technology, not politics, was what changed" in 2012 (para. 13). Social media became increasingly ubiquitous around this time, impacting youth across countries.

Jonathan Haidt (2023), in reviewing this and other data, argued that those who identify as liberal, and particularly liberal women, have the highest rates of mental illness, especially among the young. Haidt argued that this data supports the views he and Greg Lukianoff presented in 2018 in *The Coddling of the American Mind.* In particular, they argued that much of the progressive thinking encouraged on college campuses reflected a form of "reverse CBT" (Haidt, 2023, para. 3). The support of emotional reasoning, black and white thinking, and other forms of cognitive distortions promote an external locus of control and increase the perception of the world as an unfriendly place locked in a battle between good and evil people. These ideas compose the thrust of Lukianoff and Haidt's (2018) theory of what is happening for young people in the US. Haidt (2023) considered the external locus of control resulting from these distortions a primary factor affecting youth mental health, describing liberal girls in particular but all youth broadly since 2010 as having an increasingly external locus of control. He connected this to the rise of online communities like Tumblr, 4Chan, and Twitter, wherein an emphasis on non-normative identities grew and a conception of identities as fragile and words as violent, at least on Tumblr and Twitter, fomented—similar to Goldberg's (2023) observation about the rise of social media in 2012.

Lukianoff and Haidt (2018) do not argue for the exact inverse of Gimbrone et al. (2022). While Gimbrone et al. appeal to external reality for worsening liberal mental health and psychic reality for protected conservative mental health, Lukianoff and Haidt essentially appeal to psychic reality in both cases—the way one views the facts is what is either pathogenic or salutary. Despite deploying Cognitive Behavioral Therapy to explain these matters, it seems remarkable that they show a greater attention to psychic reality than do forms of psychoanalysis focused on adaptation to external reality or the adaptation of reality to the fantasy of the ego. The fantasm that structures the psyche causes numerous torsions of information in the space between percept and conscious thought. This does not dismiss the importance of the supposedly external world, but it does suggest that the fantasies that allow the social link to operate may be cultivated in ways consistent with psychoanalytic ethics or not.

One of the specific concerns that Lukianoff and Haidt (2018) raise is the splitting of the social world into purely "good" and purely "bad" elements, creating a two-dimensional virtual reality in which every person occupies a good or bad pole along various axes, such as oppressor/oppressed. Similar to the Oresteian and Stigmatic solutions to the social link failing to bind *jouissance*, this strategy also reflects a purification of the pleasure ego, an operation required to manage unbound *jouissance*. It also reflects a hostility to ambiguity that is entirely inconsistent with the core principles of psychoanalysis, such as the overdetermination of behavior (including mental behavior) and the calling into question of the subject's implication in its fantasy. With respect to the latter, it is also remarkable that Lukianoff and Haidt identify the reification of language's effects as harmful in itself, such that language can become "violence," as another problematic development in social discourse. Considering the imaginification of discourse as a result of the increasing dominance of the consumerist discourse, the valorization of the image in social media, and the failure of the Name of the Father to fully instate the symbolic, it perhaps should not be surprising that language takes on the value of the act. Without a clear symbolic network governing the social link, imaginary aggressivity comes to occupy all relations that are not based upon specular mirroring and similarity. The difference that characterizes the symbolic, in its series of oppositions between signifiers, drops away. When language becomes violence, it becomes increasingly impossible to engage in any dispute of ideas as every disagreement becomes a threat to the clarity of the mirror image. These examples illustrate that the fantasm is directly connected to the sociopolitical environment.

In fact, Glynos and Stavrakakis (2008) delineated four positions of subjectivity based on their accounting of the fantasy. They split these four positions across two axes; the first axis is the *social-political* (based on the subject's relation to social identity) and the second is the *ideological-ethical* (based on "the *mode* of the subject's engagement with…norms" [p. 265]). Their use of language in characterizing these subjective positions makes unclear whether what they have in mind—in Lacan's (1986/1992) terminology following Kant, the *Wohl* or the *Gute*. Kant (1788/2004) distinguished between the two terms by the fact that *Wohl* is associated with pleasure or pain where *Gute* is related to the Good. Lacan (1986/1992) related the *Wohl*, social well-being, to the pleasure principle that governs the level of the *Vorstellungen*, or mental representations. The *Gute* is therefore beyond the pleasure principle and pertains not to the *Sachevorstellungen* or thing-presentations but to *das Ding*, the Thing that Lacan theorized at the center of the subjective universe. To say it is not clear which Glynos and Stavrakakis (2008) have in mind is to observe that the language they use does not clearly reflect whether the social weal or subjective Good is at stake.

Nevertheless, Glynos and Stavrakakis's (2008) account provides some important grounding points that can be utilized in a theorization that goes beyond weal. What they call the *social* subject follows the regulation of societal norms as "taken for granted" while what they call the *political* subject has "contested or defended" such societal norms (p. 264). Notably, in the extended discussion after this statement, the "defended" portion drops off, implicitly privileging the *political* subject as always occupying a progressive position. Thus, social and political subjects are oriented to either the unquestioned following or contesting/defending of social norms. In addition to this axis, the authors identify the subject whose engagement with social norms is "mediated in a phallic mode," that is, by a phallic fantasy, as an *ideological* subject in contrast to the "non-phallic enjoyment" of the *ethical* subject (p. 265). They identify the phallic mode of the ideological subject as connected to "the subjects' aversion to ambiguity," which is related to the "total rejection or total embrace" of their leaders and is predicated on an "overinvestment in an ideal or norm" (p. 265). What is remarkable about this characterization is that, while their analysis still applies to the nationalism they targeted in 2008, these descriptions equally describe a significant portion of the political left in the US some 15 years later, a reflection of the increasing polarization that has compromised the social link. The "subjects' aversion to ambiguity," "total rejection or total embrace" of public figures, and totalizing tendencies are fairly apt descriptions of the electorate on both sides of the aisle in an affectively polarized society like the US. Because this action is a purification of the pleasure ego, it is inherently on the side of pleasure and inherently on the side of *Wohl*, regardless of whether Glynos and Stavrakakis would class such subjectivity as social or political. *Jouissance* is projected onto the other in such a way that it is at least temporarily bound in a social link that has failed to address it otherwise. In this way, mainstream political discourse in the US has been increasingly overtaken by, and productive of, what Glynos and Stavrakakis would call ideological subjectivities, of the left as well as the right.

Glynos and Stavrakakis's (2008) treat political life as regulated by the fantasy, such that "fantasy can be understood as a way of mediating the subject's relation to the norms and ideals governing a social or political practice" (p. 265). This raises a question for them, wherein they tentatively draw a distinction between collective and individual fantasies. This again summons the idea of a Durkheimian "collective consciousness." Lacan (1998/2017) rejected this idea, at least on its face, but also affirmed the interdependence of the subject and discourse. Lacan's (2011/2018) placement of discourse in the context of bodily *jouissance* renders attempts to separate the individual and the collective suspect from a Lacanian perspective, something Glynos and Stavrakakis (2008) seem to acknowledge when they state that "even if there are good heuristic reasons for drawing a distinction between individual and collectively shared fantasies, the conceptual implications—both theoretical and methodological—demand careful attention" (p. 270).

To pay such careful attention, one might notice that the relationship between the individual and the collective is at the center of the social-political axis of Glynos and Stavrakakis (2008). This axis seems to split subjectivity into either accepting social norms (social) or disputing them (political). Revisiting Freud's (1930) theoretical construction of the tension between the individual and civilization may help in making sense of the individual-collective problem.

Freud (1930) articulated this individual-collective tension with a uniqueness often overlooked. Despite the frequent association of Freud's account of social structure with Hobbes' anthropology, the equivalence drawn between them flattens out Freud's ideas in misleading and counterproductive ways (Kaye, 1991). Indeed, Kaye argued that to interpret Freud in a Hobbesian way, focusing only on the *"homo homini lupus"* that Freud (1930, p. 111) endorsed, leads to an oversimplified notion of Freud as seeing humans as essentially asocial actors and society as essentially a force of oppression. This negates the ambivalence central to Freud's thought, such that humans have complex and contradictory motivations. Indeed, even Freud's (1930) statement on the fundamentally lupine nature of humanity contains the dialectic that the other is "not only a potential helper or sexual object, but also someone who tempts them to satisfy their aggressiveness on him" (p. 111), that is, that the other may be the object of multiple and conflicting drive aims.

Without this central ambivalence within the subject, the tension between individual and civilization becomes one in which the individual contains only asocial drive aims (rather than an admixture of social and asocial aims) and civilization is the bulwark of stability (Kaye, 1991). Kaye viewed this false dichotomy as leading to a choice between "the necessity of conformity to cultural constraints, which we associate with the Parsonians, or the desire for instinctual liberation from cultural oppression, which we associate with the Frankfurt School and the cultural revolutionaries of the 1960s" (p. 91). Indeed, Kaye objected to the confusion of repression with suppression or oppression, a common slip in the English language where all three terms are more or less interchangeable in the political realm—one might repress dissent, oppress a people, or suppress a rival political movement, all with relatively similar intent and outcome. This leads to a dichotomous understanding of psychic repression as akin to social oppression, therefore placing liberatory struggle on the side of the drive against an oppressive social order. Kaye argued that both of what he considered the Parsonian and Frankfurtian perspectives fall into the trap of "suppressing its contradictory counterpart" (Kaye, 1991, p. 91).

If Freudian theory necessitates a more complex picture of the individual than a simplified individual-vs.-collective image presents, it is because the individual is the seat of both the drive and the repressing force of the censor. The interface between individual and collective fantasies that Glynos and Stavrakakis (2008) deliberate is a matter of the integration/regulation combination that the social link comprises. The individual fantasy is neither constitutive of nor resulting from whatever could be called a collective fantasy. Indeed, there is no such thing as a collective fantasy, as there is no collective subject to fantasize. There is only a discourse that tends to produce a certain overlapping series of fantasies, or to produce a certain quality of fantasmatic production.

While the adoption of political identities—on the right or left—is not in the same category as youth mental health at the level of social sensibilities, it does have an implication for youth mental health (Gimbrone et al., 2022). Moreover, the functions of polarization, which is concomitant with the conflation of social and political identities (Boxell et al., 2021), serve a nexus of interests: the interests of politicians seeking to create reliable market segments in the voting public, the interests of state and non-state actors in accelerating social disintegration in the US, and the interest of youth in finding some method of binding *jouissance*. All of this contributes to a broad cultural milieu that, despite being fractious to the point of political violence, finds various groups in agreement with the rejection of the ambiguity central to psychoanalytic ethics and the not-all related to non-phallic enjoyment that Glynos and Stavrakakis (2008) identify with ethical subjectivity.

As a counterpoint to the rejection of ambiguity, one might examine the film *The Starling Girl* (Parmet, 2023). The film follows the story of Jem Starling, a 17-year-old girl growing up in a conservative religious home that shuns the worldly, the bodily, and enjoyment. Jem's parents steer her toward courtship with a young man in her church with whom she is demonstrably incompatible. In the course of the film, she comes to be sexually involved with Owen, the 28-year-old married youth pastor who has recently returned from a mission trip to Puerto Rico. While an unambiguous narrative would elicit disgust at the youth pastor's exploitation of Jem—and this perspective is certainly taken at moments—Parmet sought explicitly to portray the ambivalence and complexity of the relationship, such that when the youth pastor invites Jem to run away with him to Puerto Rico to start a new life away from the punitive religious community, it is difficult not to see this from Jem's perspective as an opportunity.

Notably, the film ultimately does not condemn Owen as an unmitigated monster, nor does it excuse his behavior; neither does it show Jem in the light of a traumatized victim, although there are certainly elements of this. Instead, Parmet (2023) explicitly and intentionally stayed close to Jem's perspective and strove to portray all the characters—including Owen—as understandable humans, and to show that "patriarchal systems are harmful to everyone, not just women" (Reed, 2023, para. 7). This perspective allows for Jem to have greater autonomy; when her community presses her to confess in public for her "sin," she is clearly conflicted on the matter for many reasons. When she decides to run away with Owen, she is clearly making a decision to exit, in some form, the patriarchal community that forbade bodily enjoyment, even if this involved another form of problematic relationship. Nonetheless, her autonomous decision begat a final decision for autonomy, with Jem traveling alone in the end, to a place of happiness from her family's past, visiting a non-patriarchal version of her familial history. The ending suggests a greater connection to family, to God, and to herself than was possible in what Glynos and Stavrakakis (2008) might call the "patriarchal social logic" of her community (p. 264).

This highly nuanced examination of Jem's experience is incredibly rare in a discourse increasingly inclined to polar extremes. Were Jem, as an adult, to see an analyst or therapist, the course of treatment would likely vary widely depending on whether the analyst or therapist was capable of maintaining space for ambivalence. Many of my supervisees over the years have had a tendency to apply socially sanctioned language onto patients' experiences, such as referring to their pasts as "traumatic" when the patient has not used such language. This is not to say that events were not deeply emotionally disturbing, but to note that how each speaking being narrates its own experience is fundamental to psychoanalytic work, without trying to apply terms related only to the *Wohl* to such experiences.

Ultimately, the collapse of ambiguity is perhaps the simplest condensation of this problem related to the youth mental health crisis. Without initiation rites capable of binding *jouissance* with nuance, and in the context of the consumerist discourse's suppression of desire—which is the defense against *jouissance*—youth (and not only youth) are left with only rudimentary tools for binding *jouissance* and moving through life in ways not replete with suffering. The elimination of ambiguity, the ability to answer every question with a black-and-white response, and ultimately to provide meaning to every event is characteristic of a religion in Lacan's (2005/2013) view. In this sense, the political polarization of contemporary U.S. society reflects a certain religious moment that poses a significant threat to psychoanalysis, which is predicated on ambiguity and ambivalence. Without psychoanalysts protecting their own moderation and actively working against their own polarization, psychoanalysis risks falling into one more social lever of power serving at the hands of the most zealous true believers.

References

Boxell, L., Gentzkow, M., & Shapiro, J. M. (2021). Cross-country trends in affective polarization [Working Paper]. *National Bureau of Economic Research*. www.nber.org/system/files/working_papers/w26669/w26669.pdf.

Chinni, D. & Stamm, S. (2023, October 23). Grand Old Party: How aging makes you more conservative. *The Wall Street Journal*. www.wsj.com/politics/elections/grand-old-party-how-aging-makes-you-more-conservative-8b2515b0.

Desilver, D. (2022, March 10). The polarization in today's Congress has roots that go back decades. Pew Research Center. www.pewresearch.org/short-reads/2022/03/10/the-polarization-in-todays-congress-has-roots-that-go-back-decades/.

Dugin, A. (1997). *Foundations of geopolitics*. Arktogeja.

Dunlop, J. B. (2004). Aleksandr Dugin's Foundations of Geopolitics. *Demokratizatsiya (Washington, D.C.)*, 12(1), 41–57.

Duverger, M. (1972). *Party politics and pressure groups; a comparative introduction*. Crowell.

Gimbrone, C., Bates, L. M., Prins, S. J., & Keyes, K. M. (2022). The politics of depression: Diverging trends in internalizing symptoms among US adolescents by political beliefs. *SSM – Mental Health*, 2, 100043. doi:10.1016/j.ssmmh.2021.100043.

Glynos, J. & Stavrakakis, Y. (2008). Lacan and political subjectivity: Fantasy and enjoyment in psychoanalysis and political theory. *Critical Psychology (Lawrence & Wishart)*, 24(1), 256–274. doi:10.1057/sub.2008.23.

Goldberg, M. (2023, February 24). Don't let politics cloud your view of what's going on with teens and depression. *The New York Times*. www.nytimes.com/2023/02/24/opinion/social-media-and-teen-depression.html.

Haidt, J. (2023, March 9). Why the mental health of liberal girls sank first and fastest. *After Babel*. https://jonathanhaidt.substack.com/p/mental-health-liberal-girls.

Kant, I. (2004). *Critique of practical reason*. (T. K. Abbott, Trans.). Project Gutenberg. www.gutenberg.org/files/5683/5683-h/5683-h.htm (Original work published 1788.)

Kaye, H. L. (1991). A false convergence: Freud and the Hobbesian problem of order. *Sociological Theory*, 9(1), 87–105. doi:10.2307/201875.

Lacan, J. (1992). *The Ethics of Psychoanalysis* (J. A. Miller, Ed., D. Porter, Trans.). W. W. Norton & Co. (Original work published 1986.)

Lacan, J. (2013). *The triumph of religion: Preceded by discourse to Catholics*. (B. Fink, Trans.). Malden, MA: Polity Press. (Original work published 2005.)

Lukianoff, G. & Haidt, J. (2018). *The coddling of the American mind: How good intentions and bad ideas are setting up a generation for failure*. Penguin Books.

McCoy, J. & Press, B. (2022). What happens when democracies become perniciously polarized?Carnegie Endowment for International Peace. https://carnegieendowment.org/2022/01/18/what-happens-when-democracies-become-perniciously-polarized.

Medina, A. (2023, August 7). Gen Z voted at a higher rate in 2022 than previous generations in their first midterm election. Center for Information and Research on Civic Learning and Engagement. https://circle.tufts.edu/latest-research/gen-z-voted-higher-rate-2022-previous-generations-their-first-midterm-election.

Parker, K., Graf, N., & Igielnik, R. (2019, January 17). Generation Z looks a lot like Millennials on key social and political issues. Pew Research Center. www.pewresearch.org/social-trends/2019/01/17/generation-z-looks-a-lot-like-millennials-on-key-social-and-political-issues.

Parmet, L. (2023). *The starling girl* [film]. 2AM.

Reed, C. (2023, May 17). A Conversation With Laurel Parmet (THE STARLING GIRL). *Hammer to Nail*. www.hammertonail.com/interviews/laurel-parmet.

Roth, A. & Farrer, M. (2022, August 21). Daughter of Putin ally Alexander Dugin killed by car bomb in Moscow. *The Guardian*. www.theguardian.com/world/2022/aug/21/daughter-of-putin-ally-alexander-dugin-killed-in-car-bomb-in-moscow-reports.

S. Rep. No. 116-XX. (2019). www.intelligence.senate.gov/sites/default/files/documents/Report_Volume2.pdf.

Sahoo, N. (2020). Mounting majoritarianism and political polarization in India. In T. Carothers & A. O'Donohue (Eds), *Political Polarization in South and Southeast*

Asia: Old Divisions, New Dangers, pp. 9–24. Carnegie Endowment for International Peace. https://carnegieendowment.org/files/Political_Polarization_RPT_FINAL1.pdf.

Stuenkel, O. (2021). Brazil's polarization and democratic risks. In T. Carothers & A. E. Feldmann (Eds), *Divisive Politics and Democratic Dangers in Latin America*, pp. 8–12. Carnegie Endowment for International Peace. https://carnegieendowm ent.org/files/Carothers_Feldmann_Polarization_in_Latin_America_final1.pdf.

Part IV
Psychoanalysis in Society

10 Crooked Cures

The collapse of civil religion has hollowed out the foundation of society, eroding the shared ego ideals that could coordinate social behavior and provide the necessary substrate for social integration. This has weakened the social link and made it liable to collapse at smaller and smaller provocations. The proliferation of the fifth, consumerist discourse has chipped away at the prohibitions of society, turning transgression to profit and promoting a social link predicated almost entirely upon the image, in politics as well as economics. This has led to a moment when the most radical transgression available is to reject the hedonistic system on casters altogether, to respond to the imperative to enjoy with anhedonia and depression. On top of these two highly erosive features of contemporary U.S. society is the Internet, and especially social media. These have further destabilized central ego identifications that could bind society together. Rather, they introduce a plethora of identifications that splinter rather than unify, and which also are heavily reliant upon the image as the most important identity feature, whether through image-based social media interactions or image-based political organization.

All of this has led to a situation where rites of initiation are increasingly absent for youth. Without integrating and regulating functions to govern entrance into broader society, youth are left with a handful of options for managing the *jouissance* that never became bound within the social link, all with implications for the youth mental health crisis. One possibility is that, without recourse to community, the body of the novice becomes the grounds of a struggle with the Other, where a lack must be inscribed at all costs. *Jouissance* appears in the form of depression that rejects the super-ego's imperative for enjoyment and is controlled and bound through maneuvers such as Non-Suicidal Self-Injury, Suicidal Thoughts and Behaviors, or other sense-based delimitations on the Other's *jouissance*. The relationship between these phenomena and the youth mental health crisis is the most clear and direct, as these symptoms are tracked in descriptive fashion in much of population health surveillance of youth in the US.

A second possible resolution to the failure of initiation rites, and one that has another clear bearing on the mental health crisis, is the assumption of

DOI: 10.4324/9781032666334-15

psychiatric diagnoses as a form of symbolic nomination. This nomination provides both the integrating and regulating functions of the social link, providing induction into a community (often largely online) and a set of expected behaviors. The expected behaviors often do not include change-oriented treatment but an embrace of no longer "masking" symptoms, an acceptance of the physiological immutability of one's *jouissance* such that it would be more damaging to change it, and a performance of psychiatric and psychotherapeutic treatment as a way of validating the nomination rather than changing the diagnosis. This psychiatric nomination occurs in settings from outpatient therapy to inpatient psychiatric treatment. Because this assumption of nomination entails a different relationship to one's symptom—a belief in it from an imaginary perspective—the field of mental health is not adequately prepared for handling the use of its apparatus as a suppletion of the Name of the Father.

A third possibility for addressing the lack of social integration and regulation is assumption of social-political identities, most often focused on imaginary identifications and polarized social relations that serve to purge the ego of *jouissance*. The integration governed by imaginary identifications is by necessity imaginary, and the regulation is the regulation of the absolute, leaving no room for ambiguity or ambivalence. One is either good or bad on the basis of one's imaginary identities.

What all three resolutions have in common is the privileging and purification of the pleasure ego. Because the most pressing concern of the strengthening of *Triebanteile* is that of *jouissance*, which the social link can no longer bind, the most expedient route of managing such *jouissance* is its expulsion outward: onto the body, onto physiological anatomy, or onto the specular image of the body politic. In each case, *jouissance* belongs to the Other, never to the subject. This buttressing of the social link is, in each case, highly precarious, requiring the incurious disposition of what Lacan (1966/2006) called "the beautiful soul," "who does not recognize his very reason for being in the disorder he denounces in the world" (p. 233). Such subjective organization requires an avoidance of any question of its role in its own positionality, hence the aversion of ambiguity from these subjective positions.

However, these buttresses are only partial solutions. Even in the case of the assumption of image-based politics, *jouissance* does not disappear and mental health concerns increase. This raises an important question of how neurosis and group formation function within psychoanalysis, as one might expect a resolution of unbound *jouissance* to reduce psychic suffering.

In Freud's (1921) view, neurosis, as a failure in the social regulation of forbidden impulses, is antithetical to group structure. Neurosis renders the neurotic "asocial and should remove him from the usual group formations," and he considered it the case "that a neurosis has the same disintegrating effect upon a group as being in love" (p. 142). The individualistic results of malaise and of the assumption of diagnosis as a nomination can be considered forms of neurosis, in this narrow sense, which likely best fits with Lacan's more general elaborations of neurosis. However, Freud viewed religion as consequential precisely as a method of supplementing the repression of forbidden impulses. As he described in *The Future of an Illusion*, people's "acceptance of the universal neurosis [religion] spares them the task of constructing a personal one" (Freud, 1927, p. 44). For Freud, then, religion acts as the "universal obsessional neurosis of humanity" (p. 43). It reinforces the prohibitions that are weak in neurosis, such that those who are religious are less likely to experience neurosis than those who are not—a point Freud (1921) was willing to concede despite his own unbelief.

It is in this capacity as a replacement for personal neurosis that Freud characterized religions as *Schiefheilungen*, or "crooked cures" (p. 142). Although *Schiefheilungen* is a *hapax legomenon* in Freud's *oeuvre*, religion's role as a crooked cure is a core component of Freud's conception of religion.[1] However, he also identified additional components of religion—not only the obsessional strictures they place upon their members, but that they entail "a system of wishful illusions together with a disavowal of reality" (Freud, 1927, p. 43).

This fuller definition of religion includes three elements: reinforcing prohibitions, a system of wishful illusions, and the disavowal of reality. This provides a richer context in which to consider how such "crooked cures" may look today. The prohibitive role played by religion is precisely that which has been eroded by consumerist discourse. This renders the grounds for religion, by Freud's definition, much more fragile and difficult to cultivate as the prohibitions by such groups no longer carry the weight of a reinforcement of social prohibition. Strikingly, more Americans get their guidance on moral issues from common sense than from religion or any other source (Pew Research Center, 2015). This might be less true among tight-knit religious communities, wherein the community exists largely unto itself, without as much exposure to diversity such as in public schools. This leaves less tight-knit communities with religions largely defined by the stories they tell. Whether such stories are illusions and/or disavowals of reality is more difficult to say.

Nonetheless, what is striking is the way in which the assumption of image-based politics seems to serve a quasi-religious function. Although prohibitions may seem to be absent in such cases—that is, that such groups do not police the behavior of their own members very strictly—one must recall that *jouissance* in such groups is consistently displaced onto the Other. Because of this, the prohibitions promulgated by such groups are directed at their ideological rivals, still included in some sense but only as applied to others. This is clear in the ways that partisan commentators almost always forgive the mistakes of their favored political leaders while castigating identical failures among those against whom they campaign. Is it fair, then, to consider political ideologies as religions?

Freud (1921) believed the social link mediated by religion was already fading in his time. His view was that the overall decrease in religious intolerance in Europe did not reflect an improvement in human society but "the undeniable weakening of religious feelings and the libidinal ties which depend upon them" (pp. 98–99). At least as a factor of intolerance, Freud viewed organizing principles generally as an equivalent to religion, observing that:

> If another group tie takes the place of the religious one—and the socialistic tie seems to be succeeding in doing so–then there will be the same intolerance towards outsiders as in the age of the Wars of Religion; and if differences between scientific opinions could ever attain a similar significance for groups, the same result would again be repeated with this new motivation.
>
> (p. 99)

Thus, intolerance toward outside groups is mediated by the strength of the in-group libidinal tie. This libidinal tie has to do with both the investment of the group ego ideal as well as the regulation following therein—and it is the regulation that governs intolerance. While certain sects of religion in the world continue to reflect this form of intolerance, including violent and murderous reactions to blasphemy and heresy, religions largely do not engage in such violence in the US, arguably because of religions' weakness as a social link in this society. Nevertheless, intolerance appears to be on the rise in the form of political polarization.

Freud's concept of *Schiefheilung* has been carried forward only haltingly in analytic writing; for example, Bohleber (1992) noted that other ideological communities, in addition to religion, might serve the purpose of a *Schiefheilung*, sparing the individual a neurotic torsion. Indeed, the primary use of *Schiefheilungen* appears in connection with analyses of authoritarianism and especially antisemitism (see Brockhaus, 2022; Claussen, 1987; Schneider, 2022).

Following these theoretical developments, one might easily imagine how right-wing nationalism could be a religious movement of sorts. In many ways, the Trumpism that was ushered into public discourse in 2015 is only the logical conclusion of the breakdown of the social link. Trump offered a picture of the primal father second to no other political figure in the United States. The rules did not apply to him ($\exists x \bar{\Phi} \bar{x}$), his sexual behavior was uninhibited (*The New York Times*, 2016), pseudo-incestuous (see Rahman, 2023), and he presented the sort of imposing paternal image that worried critics about his authoritarian intentions. In 1975, Robert Bellah (1975/1992) envisioned the concerns that would arise with a figure like Trump, noting that:

> It is questionable whether a "return" to inherited ethnic and religious identities, at least among the more privileged white groups, would be

particularly healthy. A return to primordial loyalties in the face of cultural and social breakdown can be defensive, based more on fear than joyous reaffirmation. Where the motive is the protection of one's own property and privilege against the threat of other competing groups, the political implications can be quite serious. One man's "cultural pluralism" can then become another man's "nativism," with all the classic elements of violence and repression that that entails.

(p. 109–110)

The "return to primordial loyalties in the face of cultural and social breakdown" is nowhere laid more bare than in the slogan *Make America Great Again*. This is not a simple reactionary response of the privileged in the face of social progress; Trump's behavior is his embodiment of what has been decreasingly available in U.S. society: a viable ego ideal. When voters say that Donald Trump "tells it like it is" (see Markovits, 2016), this seems to be less a concern with what "it" actually "is" (i.e., something like the truth) and more a response to the perpetual spin and avoidance tactics typical of traditional politicians who are infamous for never answering a question. Trump's clear stances, however mercurial and effervescent, provide the illusion of a strong paternal figure capable of making the world right. In this sense, Trump's movement fits some Freudian notions of religion, such as providing wishful illusions that distort reality and supporting a group rather than individual neurosis in the form of *jouissance* becoming bound to events on the national stage in a way shared by group members. However, it perhaps most importantly includes the renewal of the parental complex, which Freud (1910) argued was religion's role. Just as the helpless infant could rely upon its parents to protect and care for it, the adult, when faced with helplessness, invests in ideals that can protect it in the same way. This seems to be the crucial element of authoritarianism, as it was in Freud's (1921) analysis when he considered the role of the group leader as an introjected ego ideal, the replacement of identification with the Father.

Although racism and right-wing political ideas need not necessarily coincide, it seems to be an unfortunately common occurrence, particularly in contemporary U.S. politics. Some analytically minded authors have focused on *jouissance* as the key to understanding racism (e.g., Hook, 2021), which may be true in part. However, I believe this significantly neglects aspects of mass psychology involved in racism, which is necessarily a phenomenon of social groups and not of individuals. In this respect, Declercq (2006) was correct when he argued that "one of the consequences of Lacan's axiom concerning the absence of a sexual relationship is that libidinal enjoyment does not create a bond between subjects. Nor does it have group-formative effects" (p. 75). Hook (2021) traced the theory of racism as a form of *jouissance* to Lacan's (1974/1990) *Television* interview, which took place in 1973, wherein, in response to a question regarding his prediction of increasing racism, Lacan stated:

With our *jouissance* going off the track, only the Other is able to mark its position, but only insofar as we are separated from this Other. Whence certain fantasies—unheard of before the melting pot.

Leaving this Other to his own mode of *jouissance*, that would only be possible by not imposing our own on him, by not thinking of him as underdeveloped.

Given, too, the precariousness of our own mode, which from now on takes its bearings from the ideal of an overcoming [*plus-de-jouir*], which is, in fact, no longer expressed in any other way, how can one hope that the empty forms of humanhysterianism [*humanitairerie*] disguising our extortions can continue to last?

(pp. 32–33)

Hook (2021) interpreted this, following Žižek, as an expression of the theory of stolen *jouissance* as the heart of racism. In other words, racism is based upon an experience of *jouissance* as stolen by the Other. In his words, "racism, then…is not most fundamentally about psychological rivalries, or about the need to displace onto the other what one disavows about one's self. Racism is instead to be understood as a response to the 'real' of enjoyment" (p. 44). From Hook's perspective, this seems to be a more attractive explanation than "the familiar psychodynamic idea of racism-as-projection" (p. 44). Nevertheless, this does not necessarily seem to fit with Lacan's (1974/1990) statement. The *Television* interview occurred in 1973, not long after his 1972 Milan discourse. The reference to *jouissance* going off the track seems to refer to the impacts of the capitalist discourse, which I have also called the consumer discourse, discussed in Chapter 5. The Other is no longer capable of delimiting *jouissance* except through separation from it. From this perspective, Lacan appears to be arguing that modern, multicultural societies operating from a modern, consumerist discourse create a novel ground for new fantasies to form based on an imaginary otherness. However, Lacan did not reference a stolen *jouissance* but an imposed *jouissance*. Racism, for Lacan, appears to be connected to *jouissance* in the sense that the Other is perceived to have a different *jouissance* that must, in fact, be corrected. What is especially remarkable here is that differing regimes of *jouissance* seem to imply not an individualistic fantasy of stolen *jouissance* but a product of social regulation being enforced upon another, which requires a group identification.

With this in mind, I believe it is more appropriate to consider what is often missing in *jouissance*-centered accounts: the fundamental role of group psychology in Freud's (1921) sense, and in particular the role of race as an ideal that binds groups together through identification. The use of race as an ideal is occurs in both socially beneficial as well as socially pernicious ways, just as religion might function in either way. In some cases, racial identification might serve to strengthen the ties of a community that might otherwise struggle to coordinate behavior in the face of a hostile environment—for example, immigrant communities facing discriminatory practices from a host culture might be able to obtain more equitable treatment by organizing and advocating as a group. However, such identifications may also serve inimical causes as well, such as white nationalism in the US or race-based violence across the globe.

How group identifications might result in very different outcomes—in socially salutary or pernicious outcomes—remains unclear unless one takes Lacan's (1974/1990) comments in the context of his broader work. Lacan (1966/2006, 1967) at times characterized the group formations that Freud (1921) described in his *Group Psychology* as predicated on imaginary identifications. Of such identifications, Lacan (1966/2006) stated:

> At the very least, we can say that these effects [of imaginary identification] do not foster discussion, which is at the root of all scientific progress. Identification with the image that gives the group its ideal—which is here the image of sufficiency incarnate—certainly founds, as Freud showed in a decisive schema, the communion of the group, but it is precisely at the expense of all articulate communication. Hostile tension is even constitutive of individual-to-individual relations in it.
>
> This is what the euphemism that is customary in the milieu quite validly recognizes with the expression "the narcissism of minor differences," which I will translate in more direct terms as "conformist terror."
>
> (pp. 409–410)

Lacan's take here is clear: Imaginary identification fosters a sense of group solidarity that enforces conformist terror on those who are different or are outsiders. In cases of group formation by imaginary identification, such outcomes seem reliably distinct compared to outcomes of identification predicated on a symbolic ego ideal. This is because the symbolic is predicated on difference rather than similarity, and it contains a signifier of its own lack (S[$\cancel{A}$]). Without the S($\cancel{A}$), the smoothness of the image is all that is left.

This formulation creates the possibility to extend the discussion beyond theories of racism to include the image-based politics that dominate both the political right and left in the US today. This image-based world is pertinent to Soler's (2018) observation of the "subjective context," at least in France. She noted that:

> the symbolic had changed, where the unifying semblants of discourse that once allowed for the compensation of the shortcomings of the Other are no more, where the semblant of the father no long[er] holds the function of the Other of the Other....And it is the discourse of contemporary victimisation that at the level of public and political life reanimates the groanings of the traumatic moment of childhood and redoubles them.
>
> (p. 6)

This environment—found in the US as well—is one wherein the subject cannot help but view the Other as the "traumatic parent" (p. 5); Soler argued this was the parent of the S(A̸), the Other with a hole. However, the signifier of lack in the Other is only produced at the level wherein there is, at least in fantasy, an Other of the Other. It is only when desire fails that the traumatic parent emerges, the one who could eat the child alive like the Saturn of Goya's Black Paintings that adorns the French and English covers of Lacan's (1994/2020) seminar on *The Object Relation*. It is also this parent, the full one who enjoys, that confounds the distinction Soler made between lack and loss. Lack, for Soler (2018), is structural and "inherent in the one who speaks, from the fact that [they] speak" (p. 13). This is the castration imposed by language. Loss, in contrast, "has more to do with the real, and specifically the real of the body," inclusive of those bodily experiences which produce the object *a* (p. 13). It is these two together, in Soler's reading, that constitute desire.

The elimination of the signifier of lack in the Other (S[A̸]) necessarily entails the subsumption of all pain in loss and, in fact, of all being in loss, as "desire…is the only being of the subject" and desire becomes equivalent to loss without the balance of lack (Soler, 2018 p. 12). The construction of a sort of purified loss crystalizes the Other as the castrating Other, "the father who has fucked up the kid" (Lacan, 1986/1992, p. 308). Because the structural element of desire is suppressed in discourse, loss enters perception as traumatic and without necessity. It did not have to happen. This is an imaginary basis of discourse, a product of consumerism and the proliferation of the image in television and the Internet. This imaginary basis of discourse underlies the image-based discourse on the political right as well as the left. At the extreme, both political ideologies envision an ultimate correction of society through a restoration of *jouissance*, both in the sense of restoring to the subject what was lost in the past, but also and perhaps more importantly by *imposing the correct mode of* jouissance *on the Other*, in accordance with Lacan's (1974/1990) comments. The connection to racism is, in Lacan's sense, a matter of the increasing diversity of nations in the 20th and 21st centuries. In the era of the image, the same psychical mechanisms may underlie political polarization as well.

Given the structural similarity of political ideas at the extreme ends of the spectrum, one might conclude that, just as certain right-wing ideologies can function as a *Schiefheilung*, so might certain left-wing ideologies. They similarly entail a series of illusions, a way of binding *jouissance* to the Other (however familiar this theory might be in Hook's [2021] view), and a disavowal of some aspects of reality. This conclusion is not latent in Freud but manifest. Freud's (1933) commentary on Marxism is worth considering in its fullness:

> Theoretical Marxism, as realized in Russian Bolshevism, has acquired the energy and the self-contained and exclusive character of a *Weltanschauung*, but at the same time an uncanny likeness to what it is

fighting against. Although originally a portion of science and built up, in its implementation, upon science and technology, it has created a prohibition of thought which is just as ruthless as was that of religion in the past. Any critical examination of Marxist theory is forbidden, doubts of its correctness are punished in the same way as heresy was once punished by the Catholic Church. The writings of Marx have taken the place of the Bible and the Koran as a source of revelation, although they would seem to be no freer from contradictions and obscurities than those older sacred books.

And although practical Marxism has mercilessly cleared away all idealistic systems and illusions, it has itself developed illusions which are no less questionable and unprovable than the earlier ones. It hopes in the course of a few generations so to alter human nature that people will live together almost without friction in the new order of society.... Meanwhile it shifts elsewhere the instinctual restrictions which are essential in society; it diverts the aggressive tendencies which threaten all human communities to the outside and finds support in the hostility of the poor against the rich and of the hitherto powerless against the former rulers. But a transformation of human nature such as this is highly improbable. The enthusiasm with which the mass of the people follow the Bolshevist instigation at present, so long as the new order is incomplete and is threatened from outside, gives no certainty for a future in which it would be fully built up and in no danger. In just the same way as religion, Bolshevism too must compensate its believers for the sufferings and deprivations of their present life by promises of a better future in which there will no longer be any unsatisfied need. This Paradise, however, is to be in this life, instituted on earth and thrown open within a foreseeable time. But we must remember that the Jews as well, whose religion knows nothing of an after-life, expected the arrival of a Messiah on earth, and that the Christian Middle Ages at many times believed that the Kingdom of God was at hand.

(pp. 179–180)

That political ideas, including the Leninist-Stalinist implementation of Marxism, can be religious in form was echoed, subtly, by Lacan (1986/ 1992) as well. He noted that communism is a continuation of "the eternal tradition of power" focused on a postponement of desire and that, despite its atheism, nonetheless relies upon the same "keeping of accounts" and a "notion of objective guilt" that mean "from a structural point of view... nothing is resolved" (pp. 318–319).

Those on the far ends of the political spectrum seem to think that religious illusions only exist on the other side of the aisle. Even psychoanalysts, who often train their focus upon the right when writing about social issues in psychoanalysis, might be missing opportunities to take a caring, critical lens to the left. Indeed, this is not merely idle theoretical speculation; for example, the Editorial Board of the *The New York Times* (2022), which is not generally viewed a conservative bastion (Spayd, 2016), expressed concerns about the ideological chilling of free speech as a problem among the progressive left. None of this is diminishes the seriousness of the problems of authoritarianism and racism on the right. These problems have received much more attention in psychoanalytic literature, however, and I believe psychoanalytic thought is capable of at least as much philosophical nuance as Dialectical Behavior Therapy, which teaches that two seemingly opposed things can be true.

The overarching matter of concern here is not score-keeping problems on the right and left; it is that polarization itself is reflective of the decay of any pretense to a civic identity that could include an array of perspectives. In this bimodal political distribution, there are traitors and patriots. The strength of such political consolidation from a psychic perspective is that, as each group positions itself opposite the other, they each become a stronger group, providing a greater degree of "crooked cure."

Left without adequate initiation into the social link, youth will adopt group identities as stopgap measures. They adopt polarized positions as new *Weltanschauungen*, conferring at least some of the benefits of religion. While suffering remains, it is a socialized suffering that occurs in the context of a metanarrative that allows for a suppression of the subject's lack.

The recurrence of religious functions in ostensibly secular politics is not necessarily problematic; humanity has embraced religion since the earliest times, during which it was largely coterminous with politics, and there is no reason to imagine that humanity would truly divest its politics of religion any time soon. However, religious fundamentalism is worth examination in any of its forms.

Lacan (2005/2013) once commented that religion—particularly the religion in which he was raised, Catholicism—would one day triumph over psychoanalysis. He predicted this because psychoanalysis subsists in the form of a question about the gap between the speaking being and its ability to cobble together a semblance and an ego; the industrial revolution and the scientific and technological consequences of it opened the subject to a much wider gap than previous centuries, as technological advancements raised many questions about meaning and significance. God became less and less central in post-Enlightenment thought, a series of revolutions destabilized the traditional political order, and theories of evolution began to displace the position of humanity at the peak of the created order. What did it all mean? In this gap, Freud constructed psychoanalysis. But, Lacan contended, religion provides answers to all forms of gap and removes all questions, and it would do the same in the future if given enough time to catch up. In the United States today, it seems Lacan may have been correct, but it is not a religion in the traditional sense that is providing answers to everything in a way that ends psychoanalysis, it is polarized political ideologies.

In considering the future of the Marxist revolution in the USSR, Freud (1933) found himself unable to meaningfully comment on whether the

Communist "experiment" would be fruitful (p. 181). What he was certain about was that "we shall still have to struggle for an incalculable time with the difficulties which the untamable character of human nature presents to every kind of social community" (p. 181). I share Freud's reservations about overly ambitious attempts at transforming humanity; while it is more plea- surable to maintain a cheerful optimism that progress inherently means moving forward and evolving positively, this historicist approach is pre- dicated on a developmentalism at odds with a Lacanian perspective. Time will tell what the outcome of recent polarization will be for youth today. If the early signs are indicators, there will be much work to do going forward.

Note

1 This idea shows up as early as 1910 in Freud's address to the Second Psychoanalytic Congress.

References

Bellah, R. (1992). *The broken covenant: American civil religion in a time of trial.* University of Chicago Press. (Original work published 1975.)

Bohleber, W. (1992). Nationalism, hatred of foreigners and antisemitism. Psychoanalytic considerations. *Psyche (Stuttgart)*, 46(8), 689–709.

Brockhaus, G. (2022). Hasspolitik – Ansteckungsangst und Abwehr. *Psyche (Stutt- gart)*, 76(7), 599–631. doi:10.21706/ps-76-7-599.

Claussen, D. (1987). Über Psychoanalyse und Antisemitismus. *Psyche (Stuttgart)*, 41(1), 1–21.

Declercq, F. (2006). Lacan on the capitalist discourse: Its consequences for libidinal enjoyment and social bonds. *Journal for the Psychoanalysis of Culture and Society*, 11(1), 74–83. doi:10.1057/palgrave.pcs.2100068.

Editorial Board of the New York Times. (2022, March 18). America has a free speech problem. *The New York Times.* www.nytimes.com/2022/03/18/opinion/cancel- culture-free-speech-poll.html.

Freud, S. (1910). The future prospects of psycho-analytic therapy. *The Standard Edi- tion of the Complete Psychological Works of Sigmund Freud* (Vol. XI), pp. 139– 152. Hogarth Press.

Freud, S. (1921). Group psychology and the analysis of the ego. *The Standard Edition of the Complete Psychological Works of Sigmund Freud* (Vol. XVIII), pp. 65–144. Hogarth Press.

Freud, S. (1927). The future of an illusion. *The Standard Edition of the Complete Psychological Works of Sigmund Freud* (Vol. XXI), pp. 1–56. Hogarth Press.

Freud, S. (1933). New introductory lectures on psycho-analysis. *The Standard Edition of the Complete Psychological Works of Sigmund Freud* (Vol. XXII), pp. 1–182. Hogarth Press.

Haidt, J. (2023, March 9). Why the mental health of liberal girls sank first and fastest. *After Babel.* https://jonathanhaidt.substack.com/p/mental-health-liberal-girls.

Hook, D. (2021). Pilfered pleasure: on racism as "the theft of enjoyment". In S. George & D. Hook (Eds), *Lacan and Race: Racism, Identity, and Psychoanalytic Theory*, pp. 35–50. Routledge.

Lacan, J. (1972). Du discours psychanalytique. In *Lacan in Italia 1953–1978 en Italie Lacan*, pp. 27–39. La Salamandra.

Lacan, J. (1990). *Television: A challenge to the psychoanalytic establishment*. J. Copjec (Ed.). (D. Hollier, R. Krauss, A. Michelson, & J. Mehlman, Trans.). W.W. Norton & Co.

Lacan, J. (1992). *The ethics of psychoanalysis*. J. A. Miller (Ed.). (R. Grigg, Trans.). W. W. Norton & Co. (Original work 1986.)

Lacan, J. (2013). *The triumph of religion: Preceded by discourse to Catholics*. (B. Fink, Trans.). Polity Press. (Original work published 2005.)

Lacan, J. (2020). *The object relation: The seminar of Jacques Lacan, Book* IV. J. A. Miller (Ed.). (A. R. Price, Trans.). Polity Press. (Original work published 1994.)

Lukianoff, G. & Haidt, J. (2018). *The coddling of the American mind: How good intentions and bad ideas are setting up a generation for failure*. Penguin.

Markovits, E. (2016, March 4). Trump 'tells it like it is.' That's not necessarily a good thing for democracy. *The Washington Post*. www.washingtonpost.com/news/monkey-cage/wp/2016/03/04/trump-tells-it-like-it-is-thats-not-necessarily-a-good-thing-for-democracy.

The New York Times. (2016, October 8). Transcript: Donal Trump's taped comments about women. *The New York Times*. www.nytimes.com/2016/10/08/us/donald-trump-tape-transcript.html.

Pew Research Center. (2015). U.S. public becoming less religious [White Paper]. Pew Research Center. www.pewresearch.org/religion/wp-content/uploads/sites/7/2015/11/201.11.03_RLS_II_full_report.pdf.

Rahman, K. (2023, June 28). Exclusive: Trump made shocking comments about Ivanka, says ex-staffer. *Newsweek*. www.newsweek.com/donald-trump-ivanka-naked-sexism-miles-taylor-book-nyt-anonymous-1809187.

Schneider, V. (2022). Prüfstein der Freiheit – Psychoanalyse und Gesellschaftskritik heute. *Psyche (Stuttgart)*, 76(8), 708–719. doi:10.21706/ps-76-8-708.

Soler, C. (2018). *Humanisation? Psychoanalysis, symbolisation, and the body of the unconscious* (B. Farrow & H. D'Alascio, Trans.). Routledge.

Spayd, L. (2016, July 23). Why readers see the Times as liberal. *The New York Times*. www.nytimes.com/2016/07/24/public-editor/liz-spayd-the-new-york-times-public-editor.html.

11 Elements of an Ethical Response

In 1897, Emile Durkheim (1897/1997) published his detailed, landmark study of suicide and its causes. His ideas were remarkable for their essentially sociological nature; that is, he accounted for suicide not as a matter of individual psychology but as a *sui generis* phenomenon of society. Durkheim found two axes central to explaining suicide: integration and regulation, both related to the social bond. Integration is the inclusion of the individual within the group, with salutary effects most noticeable for groups that the individual loves, such that the individual will put the good of the group above the good of their self. Regulation, in contrast, is the axis representing the effects of society in regulating the behavioral and moral expression of individuals. In particular, regulation is the "degree to which a given group's rules and social norms were consensually clear, coherent, and shared" (Mueller et al., 2021, p. 3).

Durkheim's (1897/1997) two axes yield four categories of suicide based on the degree of presence or absence of integration and regulation. These categories include egoistic suicide, altruistic suicide, anomic suicide, and fatalistic suicide.

Egoistic suicide pertains to the dearth of integration, wherein the social bond is weakened by disintegrating forces. Principally, Durkheim (1897/1997) connected this to increased education, although insisted vehemently that knowledge itself was not the culprit of disintegration. Rather, he attributed the increase in desire for knowledge to the disorganization of religious systems, noting that "faith is not uprooted by dialectic proof; it must already be deeply shaken by other causes to be unable to withstand the shock of an argument" (p. 169). The search for knowledge as a replacement of collective systems of belief is the introduction of disintegrative danger; knowledge sought for other purposes, as a means rather than an end, is not deleterious itself.

Altruistic suicide, for Durkheim (1897/1997), is caused by a nimiety of integration; one is so integrated within the collective that suicide becomes a submission to the social good at certain moments, such as deaths of honor, deaths of those entering old age, deaths of household members upon the death of the head of house, and so on. In this case, it is not individualization

DOI: 10.4324/9781032666334-16

that severs social bonds and loosens the barriers against suicide, it is integration with the collective to the point of loosening the barriers against suicide found in the value of the individual.

In distinction from the suicidal categories of integration are the suicidal categories of regulation. The first of these, on the side of excessive control, is fatalistic suicide, a category Durkheim (1897/1997) viewed as so infrequent in his era that he devoted all of one footnote to it, simply to acknowledge the balancing of the continuum of regulation in the same way as that of integration. Perhaps this speaks of something indomitable in the human spirit.

On the other side of regulation from fatalistic suicide is anomic suicide, predicated on the insufficiency of regulation—regulation, specifically, of human desire (Durkheim, 1897/1997). For Durkheim, there is a careful balance that must be achieved between human appetite and means to achieve satisfaction of the appetite. While physiological needs may be proportionally satisfied, particularly in animals, Durkheim considered humanity's reflectiveness the cause of a divergence between physiological need and the appetite of the human person. In some ways, this presages Freud's own consideration of the drive and, later, Lacan's dialectic of desire. Durkheim observed that physiological needs have a limit in their satisfaction, yet the appetite of the human is insatiable if not confronted with limitations. Desires without limits "constantly and infinitely surpass the means at their command" (p. 247), running aground not on structural boundaries that shape and mold desire but on the radical inability of the environment to provide satisfaction of the wild appetite. With this in mind, Durkheim argued that "to pursue a goal which is by definition unattainable is to condemn oneself to a state of perpetual unhappiness" (p. 248). Because this abyssal desire is not organic, there is no endogenous method of control; the only method of regulating it is through social forces. Anomic suicide, then, is what occurs in the face of deregulation in society, specifically the loss of any moral method of directing desire within certain bounds. This might be a disaster of economic success and growth as much as a disaster in the sense of economic downturn. Any disruption of equilibrium at the individual or societal level— any dispersion of socially sanctioned regulations—may produce anomie.

Durkheim (1897/1997) identified one area in particular as productive of anomie, above and beyond any intermittent disasters or disruptions—that of industrial economics, regardless of political philosophy. Because both more conservative "orthodox economists" and the "extreme socialists" take "industrial prosperity" as their focus, they are not ultimately different with respect to their underlying construction of the world (p. 255). Any system that views the distribution of material goods as the highest form of organization shares a fundamental materialism. Such materialism leads to an environment, where:

> From top to bottom of the ladder, greed is aroused without knowing where to find ultimate foothold. Nothing can calm it, since its goal is far

beyond all it can attain. Reality seems valueless by comparison with the dreams of fevered imaginations; reality is therefore abandoned, but so too is possibility abandoned when it in turn becomes reality. A thirst arises for novelties, unfamiliar pleasures, nameless sensations, all of which lose their savor once known.

(p. 256)

This picture of a society incapable of regulating desire describes nothing better than consumerism in its fullest form, in economics as well as in politics. The twisting of the fantasy to interpret any limit or lack as a trauma reflects the way society is sandwiched between "the conjunction of a destructive and acephalous capitalism on the one side and of a power at the head of state who is powerless to curb the consequences of it, on the other" (Soler, 2018, p. 5). The Other is no longer incomplete but withholding.

The arguments of preceding chapters have cataloged the ways in which contemporary U.S. society reflects the bending of the social link around both the poles of lack in Durkheim's (1897/1997) system—too little integration, too little regulation. In the anomic sense, consumerism has eaten away at social regulation like a corrosive base, encouraging always a traversal of the limits of desire. Simultaneously, the loss of semblants of civil religion has left desiccated the integrative capacities of the social link. Layered on top of this, the technological developments and political polarization characterizing the country serve as both products of and further contributors to the reckless circuit without brakes the consumerist discourse compels subjects to traverse.

In the face of such broad, sociological forces, how could something as parochial as psychoanalysis make a difference? This question is of greater complexity than it may first seem. I believe there are two primary positive answers to this question, but a negative must first be considered.

There is a tension within psychoanalysis that is central to its character and too often unconsidered in both clinical writing as well as theoretical essays and papers analyzing social issues. This tension comes from one's interpretation of the psychoanalytical ethical position. Lacan (1986/1992), in his *Ethics* seminar, presented social conceptions of "good" and "bad," "right" and "wrong" as elements of the psyche relevant only insofar as they are "clues to that which orients the position of the subject, according to the pleasure principle, in connection with that which will never be more than representation" (p. 63). This thing that will never be more than a representation, which exists at another level, is the center of the subjective universe. Lacan identified this as *das Ding*, the Thing. The Thing, for Lacan, was related not to the *Wohl* of wellbeing but to the *Gute*, the ultimate good beyond pleasure, again relying on Kant's (1788/2004) distinction. Lacan's (1986/1992) lectures in this year of his seminar culminated, in the interpretations of some, in the ethical maxim that questions only whether one has "acted in conformity with the desire that is within you" (p. 314). This is the question he imagined falling with "the force of the Last Judgment," a question of import from a final perspective (p. 314). This is often paired with his statement in the same lecture on July 6, 1960, that "from an analytical point of view, the only thing of which one can be guilty is of having given ground relative to one's desire" (p. 319).

This emphasis on desire has at times been construed by analytic writers as an axiomatic statement of a universal ethic, that is, that none should cede desire in any case. This raises desire to the level of a categorical imperative, a term I choose intentionally and to which I will return.

Soler (2018) opposed such an elevation of desire, noting that Lacan's (1986/1992) teachings in the seventh year of his seminar seem to differ from those in his 24th year, wherein, as she put it, "he said...about psychoanalysis, that it is a practice without value, which does not mean that it is worthless but rather that it does not have recourse to any value whatsoever," (p. 23).[1] She criticized the tendencies in Lacanian circles to create values of the real or of desire, noting that Lacan himself asked "whether or not psychoanalysis was going to become the religion of desire" (p. 23).

Dany Nobus, in his 2022 *Critique of Psychoanalytic Reason*, drew pointed attention to something akin to Soler's concerns. While Soler presented Lacan's ethics having changed over the course of his seminar—from privileging desire to emptying analysis of values—Nobus gave a sharp rebuke to what he saw as a persistent and intransigent misreading of Lacan's comments in his *Ethics*. Specifically, Nobus objected to the reading of Lacan's (1986/1992) statement about "giving ground relative to one's desire" (p. 319) as anything approaching a universal ethical axiom. Instead, Lacan, in Nobus' (2022) reading, was merely observing a clinical phenomenon— neurotics, in contrast to what we typically think, feel guilty when they have *not* acted on their desire rather than the other way around. Beyond this, Nobus also objected that the argument that never giving ground on one's desire is somehow an ethical axiom:

> Could only be formulated by someone who has never had any clinical psychoanalytic experience, or whose professional and/or personal interests are extremely far removed from what is at stake in the psychoanalytic treatment of patients. Were a psychoanalyst to operate with the ethical precept that patients should consistently, if not always explicitly, be brought to the point where they can accept that the source of their happiness is always to be found in "not giving up on their desire," she or he would not only run the risk of aiding and abetting the patient to commit various (criminal) transgressions, but much more problematically he or she would also be acting upon the illusion that happiness coincides with the fulfilment [sic] (satisfaction or gratification) of desire. Were "Do not give up on your desire!" to be framed in gold above the psychoanalytic couch, the patient would not only be spending money on learning how to exchange a life of suffering for that of a

criminal, but the analyst would effectively be joining the reprehensible ranks of all those *faux* experts who cunningly take advantage of some-one's else's problems in order to enrich themselves through the sale of false hope and empty promises.

(p. 224)

Nobus' trenchant criticism highlights, with a refreshing intellectual honesty, the actual consequences of certain forms of academic thought that seem to echo around the (especially Lacanian) psychoanalytic community.

There are two important angles to consider alongside Nobus' (2022) two objections. First, with respect to his appeal to the absence of "any kind of textual evidence" for the interpretation of Lacan's comments as axiomatic, one can easily investigate this directly, although Nobus does not give extended attention to this (p. 224). For example, in describing the analyst's desire on June 22, 1960, Lacan (1986/1992) differentiates the analyst's desire from the analysand's to the degree it is an "experienced desire," which in part means that the analyst does not "remain in the trap that is the desire to reduce" the drive to instinct, that is, to something satisfiable (p. 301). Moreover, should the analyst take such a stance, "the subject can achieve nothing but some form of psychosis or perversion," and of the idea that the analyst could somehow bring the analysand to a point of harmony between nature and culture in this way, "one can only say of such an aspiration that it is pathetic in its naivete. And one is only surprised that it could have been formulated other than as a dead-end to be dismissed" (p. 301). Here, shortly before his comments about desire, Lacan clearly argues against the idea that the analyst might strive after satisfying either their own desire or the analysand's.

Similarly, Lacan (1986/1992) was extremely tentative about the idea of an ethics of psychoanalysis, opening the last lesson, on July 6, by stating:

"if there is an ethics of psychoanalysis—the question is an open one—it is to the extent that analysis in some way or other, no matter how minimally, offers something that is presented as a measure of our action—or it at least claims to."

(p. 311)

Lacan immediately repudiates after this the idea that psychoanalysis would eradicate all prohibition or encourage people to act on every desire, stating that he thought these ideas "had disappeared over forty years ago" (p. 312).

Even considering the larger picture of Lacan's work, the supposed call for acting in conformity with desire does not really make sense; as Nobus (2022) commented, "What Antigone teaches Lacan, during the four weeks they go on a journey together, is that the realization of one's desire does not by definition lead to happiness" (p. 224). That is, to the extent one actually approaches the Thing (which has the characteristics that would go on to become Lacan's object *a*, cause of desire), the more one is disturbed by an increasingly threatening *jouissance*. One must recall, after all, that "desire is a defense, a defense against going beyond a limit in *jouissance*," a statement which Lacan (1966/2006, p. 699) presented at a conference in Royaumont in September 1960, some months after the conclusion of his *Ethics* seminar. This is entirely consistent with Lacan's use of Kant's *Wohl* and *Gute*; the *Gute* of the Thing is what is beyond the pleasure principle, and this is unbearable. To approach it, as did Antigone, is not necessarily a matter to emulate. After all, Lacan's (1966/2006) concept of juxtaposing "Kant with Sade" is about the way in which the categorical imperative is fundamentally consistent with the sexual fetishism to which the Marquis lends his name. Indeed, in considering the sadistic nature of the superego—that is, the will-to-*jouissance* that animates it—one should also consider Lacan's (1986/1992) objection that the superego "has nothing to do with the moral con-science" and "what the superego demands has nothing to do with that which we would be right in making the universal rule of our actions" (p. 310).

Lacan (1986/1992) also averred that "constructing the instincts, in making them the natural law of the realization of harmony, psychoanalysis takes on the guise of a rather disturbing alibi, of a moralizing hustle or bluff, whose dangers cannot be exaggerated" (p. 312). That is, to construe the drive—which is not biological and is not satisfiable—as identical to the instinct—which is biological and satisfiable—is a source of danger. Remarkably, he thought this so obvious to his audience he did not bother taking this train of thought any farther.

Lest this seem like mere caviling, one should consider Nobus' (2016) account of Abdoulaye Yerodia Ndombasi, the Congolese politician who spent a significant amount of time in Paris, attending Lacan's lectures and eventually becoming his "butler and right-hand man" (p. 3). In the 1990s, he returned to the Congo to support the president, at which time his speech in "a radio broadcast Yerodia…reportedly called for the merciless extermina-tion of the aggressor, which was believed to have triggered the renewed slaughter of the Congo's Tutsi ethnic minority during the late Summer and Autumn of 1998" (p. 2). Nobus (2016; 2022) highlighted that Yerodia appealed to Lacan's teaching on desire to justify his actions, including the supposed injunction never to give up on one's desire.

I believe this sort of deployment of psychoanalytic language (I won't go so far as to say discourse) to support an episode of immense violence is pre-cisely what Lacan (1986/1992) had in mind when he said the collapse of drive and instinct is a process "whose dangers cannot be exaggerated" (p. 312). The reason for this is that once the drive is able to be satisfied in harmony with nature, there would not exist the antimony between culture and nature that Freud (1930) observed and, consequently, psychoanalysis would be beholden, after all, to genitality and "what is so imprudently linked to it, namely, adjustment to reality" (Lacan, 1986/1992, p. 293).

There would be a correct functioning of the human that psychoanalysis would then enforce in the form of a moral pedagogy. Nobus (2016) discussed the philosophical problems that arise from this, when psychoanalysis might grab the reins of power to proclaim right from wrong—power, here, in Lacan's (1986/1992) sense: "a human—far too human—power," one that says "carry on working" and "as far as desires are concerned, come back later" (pp. 314–315).

It is critical to consider this ethical dimension in psychoanalysis before considering any intervention at the level of initiation rites because what that intervention looks like will depend upon the ethics involved. The most significant risk, I believe, stems from the fact that the collapse of desire and demand in the consumerist fifth discourse is precisely the collapse of instinct and drive of which Lacan warned and submission to which psychoanalysis is not immune. In considering psychoanalysis's vulnerability to polarization and succumbing to imaginary political not-very-funhouses, one need look no further than the events in the American psychoanalytic institutes and societies in 2023.[2] Psychoanalytic clinicians, once convinced they have the absolute truth, are no safer than any other human with such convictions, however much they think themselves better prepared to sort fact from fiction.

Nobus (2016) outlined four possible approaches to the question of psychoanalytic ethics. The first, which he attributed to Jacques Derrida and René Major, is a solution involving a reconsideration of an overarching ethical system in society, first articulated as psychoanalysis integrating itself into larger ethical frameworks, and later as an injunction to such frameworks, legally and politically, to incorporate psychoanalytic knowledge into their ethical formulations. As Nobus pointed out, these two formulations of the same position are contradictory, and the more recent version leaves an unclear path forward in terms of how psychoanalysis, without taking an active role in such a process, could contribute to its integration into ethical, legal, or political fields.

The second approach to psychoanalytic ethics is the position that pushes to purge from psychoanalysis anything like an ethic. This position Nobus (2016) attributed to Jean Allouch. Allouch argued that the "ethification" of psychoanalysis would ultimately "surreptitiously [transform] its discourse into a political ideology" (Nobus, 2016, p. 10). He argued that the assumption of an ethical position does not protect one from unethical, morally damaging, or cruel behavior, as such behaviors are typically undertaken by those with a strong sense of ethics. Allouch argued, moreover, that Freud objected to the use of psychoanalysis as a form of moral education, and Lacan's statements are entirely consistent with this objection. However, Nobus rightfully points out that the stance of having no ethical conviction is itself an ethical conviction and therefore subject to internal inconsistency. Nonetheless, it is also true that the assumption that an ethical position is itself a protection against problematic behavior is inaccurate. This is not (only) because one might hold an ethical principle to which one does not adhere (i.e., not living up to one's own ethical standard) but because one's very ethical principles can conflict with other ethical principles or behaviors. One example of such a challenge is the issue of excluding certain candidates or analysts from psychoanalysis as a practice or as an institution. In other words, to exclude certain members from the community necessarily relies upon a moral judgment of their character, something to which Allouch objected. Once again, this is not an academic exercise; Allouch, and Nobus as well, discussed these ethical challenges in the context of the Amilcar Lobo Moreira affair. Lobo was a Brazilian psychoanalytic candidate who participated in governmental torture in the 1970s, and the question of his exclusion from analysis and the psychoanalytic community was a controversy for decades to follow.

The decision to exclude someone like Lobo may seem straightforward in some ways, yet the question of moral evaluation and the exclusion of certain people from analysis is quite complex. Torture may be an especially stark and clear case, but what about an analysand who presents with a symptom related to some less extreme form of sadistic pleasure, presenting specifically to address such a symptom? Should this person be refused psychoanalysis? Whose moral judgment decides where the line is regarding which behaviors are acceptable or not under such a regime? This pathway is a few steps away from tests of ideological purity, especially considering the requirement that analysts enter the field first as analysands. Even if it is not possible to eliminate the ethical from psychoanalysis to avoid such problems, these questions must be taken seriously in any account of psychoanalytic ethics.

The third approach to the ethics of psychoanalysis, which Nobus (2016) attributed to Baidou, follows Allouch's approach in critiquing ethical ideology but presents, rather than a purgation of ethics, a focus only on purging ethical ideology. However, Nobus raises again the concern that Baidou has misread Lacan's statement about giving ground on desire, leading to a misunderstanding of psychoanalytic ethics. In this case, Nobus points to the highly risky position this offers, as "a Kantian categorical imperative can justify the most extreme act of terror" (p. 14).

In contrast to these positions, Nobus (2016) described Lacan's own ambivalence about his *Ethics*, noting that in the twentieth year of his seminar, *Encore*, Lacan (1975/1998) admitted to a "not wanting to know anything about" an ethics of psychoanalysis (p. 1). For Nobus (2016), this is a sign of Lacan being "seriously dissatisfied with the results of the Ethics of Psychoanalysis" (p. 16). Instead, Nobus proposes to take Lacan's *oeuvre* in the light of his later reluctance—echoing Freud's—toward an ethics of psychoanalysis. In his view:

> The Lacanian position, if it deserves to be designated as such, does not favour an exclusion of ethics, and thus also avoids the trap of an

insidious re-emergence of ethics through the backdoor [as in Allouch's approach]. The Lacanian position neither endorses, nor rejects ethics as an operative tool for the direction of the treatment. After all, if ethics is a transformation of the Superego, it is not desirable to increase its sphere of influence, but it is equally impossible to escape it. The Lacanian position, therefore, merely acknowledges that the Superego is operative and remains indifferent to its hidden seductions.

(pp. 16–17)

With this view, Nobus sought a kind of true neutral alignment for psychoanalysis, one neither invested in purging ethics nor imposing it.

One element that strikes me as especially important that Nobus (2016) alluded to but never explicitly discussed is the tension between a universal ethic and a particular ethic. Nobus critically observed, for example, that "Badiou's ethical axioms are meant to be universal, despite the fact that every truth and every situation needs to be evaluated in its singularity" and that this axiomatic approach was "an ethical principle with universal value, equally applicable to situations within and outside the field of psycho-analysis" (p. 13). Nobus categorizes the reading of Lacan's (1986/1992) statement in his *Ethics* as a "universal ethical rule" as erroneous (Nobus, 2016, p. 13), opposing its extension as a universal axiom, owing to the consequences of such an extension. Nobus read Lacan's statement about giving ground on one's desire not as an imperative (indeed, Lacan did not write it imperatively, as Nobus correctly observed) but as a clinical observation. The context of Lacan's (1986/1992) words is instructive:

It is in an experimental form that I advance the following propositions here. Let's formulate them as paradoxes. Let's see what they sound like to analysts' ears.

I propose then that, from an analytical point of view, the only thing of which one can be guilty is of having given ground relative to one's desire.

Whether it is admissible or not in a given ethics, that proposition expresses quite well something that we observe in our experience.

(p. 319)

Notice that Lacan begins by calling this proposition "experimental," that he grounds it specifically in an "analytical point of view" (not a universal per-spective), and that the proposition only expresses something psychoanalysts observe in their clinical experience. How far from an imperative this is! Nobus (2016) called attention to this observation's relevance as a paradox, according to Lacan's introduction of it, because one typically thinks of guilt springing from having done something one wanted to do but ought not have rather than not doing something one wanted to do but ought not to have. This is the paradox.

Further insight can be found regarding Lacan's (1986/1992) commentary when considering the other half of his oft-quoted comments on desire. This second one, also from the last session in this year of the seminar, is as follows:

> It is because we know better than those who went before how to recognize the nature of desire, which is at the heart of this experience, that a reconsideration of ethics is possible, that a form of ethical judgment is possible, of a kind that gives this question the force of a Last Judgment: Have you acted in conformity with the desire that is in you?
>
> This is not an easy question to sustain. I, in fact, claim that is has never been posed with that purity elsewhere, and that *it can only be posed in the analytic context.*
>
> (p. 314, emphasis added)

Taking this pericope as a whole, Lacan clearly stated here that such an ethical question is explicitly not possible outside the context of a psychoanalysis. This already places a sharp limit on the extent to which Lacan intended his words to be taken. Why would this question only be able to be posed in the analytic context?

Two sessions before this, Lacan (1986/1992) discussed the fact that desire is central in analysis, but that the analyst's desire is an "experienced desire" that does not attempt to collapse need, demand, and desire. I believe this is why the question of whether one has acted according to one's desire, as an ethical question, can only be articulated in the context of an analysis, wherein that question is delimited in very specific ways.

In exploring *Antigone*, Lacan (1986/1992) explicitly drew on Aristotle's (ca. 335 BCE/1907) view that tragedy involves the purging of pity and fear. Making the obvious connection to psychoanalysis, Lacan (1986/1992) noted that it is by "the intervention of pity and fear, that we are purged, purified of everything of that order. And that order…is properly speaking the order of the imaginary" (p. 248). While ostensibly talking about dramatic tragedy, this also encapsulates something of the psychoanalytic process—and why else would Lacan select tragedy as a crescendo for his lecture on the *Ethics of Psychoanalysis*? This is why in his remarks on June 15, 1960, he stated that he required his audience to go through the analysis of *Antigone* with him so that such difficult ethical work "will enter your body" (p. 284). He also began his 22nd lecture, immediately after his detour on *Antigone*, by noting such a detour "was necessary so as to bring you closer to our ethics as analysts" (p. 291). Notable here again is Lacan's demarcation of the ethics he discusses first to psychoanalysis and then, even more specifically, to "our ethics *as analysts*," which is not the same as an ethic that would fully govern even the whole of an individual.

The reason that the question can only be posed within psychoanalysis is because of the ethical position of the analyst, not because of the ethical

formation of the analysand. The analyst has undergone a purging of imaginary investments such that one's desire is experienced, that is, no longer
seeks the imaginary collapse of desire and demand. The result is that "the
ethics of psychoanalysis has nothing to do with speculation about prescrip-
tions for, or the regulation of, what I have called the service of goods"
(Lacan, 1986/1992, p. 313). Lacan opposed the positioning of the analyst as
"guarantor of the possibility that a subject will in some way be able to find
happiness" as "a form of fraud" (p. 303).

These observations can be taken a few steps further. If Lacan's ethics are
not deontological (Kantian), not concerned with the ordering of goods (not
utilitarian), what sort of ethic might this be? While Lacan (1986/1992)
objected to Aristotle's conception of virtue as achieved in the golden mean,
this was in the context of considering, as Miller's chapter heading puts it,
"the demand for happiness and the promise of psychoanalysis" (p. 291). In
reality, Lacan's approach to psychoanalysis is fundamentally predicated on
the idea that something in the analysand changes as a result of the analysis
that creates a purgation of imaginary investments and institutes an experienced desire that does not fall into imaginary traps. Whether this is properly
a "virtue" may be debated, but Lacan's avoidance of a strict technicalism in
practice reflects his eschewing of Kantian imperatives, just as his rejection of
happiness as a goal of analysis reflects a refusal of utilitarianism. What
Lacan did seem to care a great deal about is the formation of the analyst. His
writing is meant not to be read but to evoke (Lacan, 1975/1998), his signifiers to be traversed (Lacan, 1973/1978), his lessons to be taken into the
body (Lacan, 1986/1992). This is the first of two directions that an ethics of
psychoanalysis must consider.

The second is that at no point did Lacan ever put forth or promulgate any
form of universal ethic (Nobus, 2016; 2022). Why it is that many commentators on Lacan seem to make the jump from Lacan's (1986/1992) commentary to a consistent psychoanalytic ethic is one question; why this ethic
is envisioned in many cases as applying outside the realm of the consulting
room is another, more abstruse question.

Taken together, one might contribute to Nobus' (2016) formulation by
suggestion that, in fact, a certain type of ethic does exist in psychoanalysis,
but it is neither one that provides guidance in a deontological or utilitarian
sense nor one that could possibly govern the world. It is one found in the
person who has undergone an analysis and pertains to the purification of
their desire. This is not inconsistent or in conflict with the notion of the *sinthome* or the idea of coming into being in the place where "it" speaks.
These are simply Lacan's other variations on the same theme.

All of this is preliminary to any consideration of the youth mental health
crisis because psychoanalysis first has to ask, without reference to the service of goods, what precisely this crisis entails. Similarly, those in the psychoanalytic community must consider whether the intervention they
propose—in any social circumstance whatsoever—is predicated on the

regulation or service of goods. It is not a problem to have social entanglements nor to take strong political positions; but these are inherently not
compatible with the role of the psychoanalyst *qua* psychoanalyst. The
deployment of psychoanalytic theory for, to borrow Freud's (1939) term,
"tendentious purposes" (p. 33) is just as distorting to psychoanalytic theory
as Freud believed such purposes were to whatever historical events might be
said to lie under the canon of holy scripture.

Most frequently, such deployments are found on the side of progressive
arguments. Perhaps this itself is progress from the days when psychoanalysis
was utilized for reactionary purposes, but the use of psychoanalysis to
advance political goals in any case raises problems (after all, people
obviously felt the use of psychoanalysis for reactionary purposes as appropriate at some point). Despite the use of Lacanian theory to formulate progressive arguments, Lacan himself was not progressive. One may read the
transcript of what happened when agitators interrupted Lacan's talk, one
part of a series of "impromptus," at Vincennes on December 3, 1969 (Lacan,
1991/2007). It is a remarkable encounter, as Lacan's response is indicative
of a very different psychoanalytic perspective than that advocated by many
psychoanalysts and psychoanalytic professionals in the US today, including
some Lacanians. Confronted repeatedly by revolutionary and Marxist
interlocutors, Lacan eventually responded to them that:

> If you had a bit of patience, and if you really wanted our impromptu to
> continue, I would tell you that, always, the revolutionary aspiration has
> only a single possible outcome—of ending up as the master's discourse.
> This is what experience has proved. What you aspire to as revolution-
> aries is a master. You will get one.... I am, like everybody is, liberal
> only to the extent that I am antiprogressive. With the caveat that I am
> caught up in a movement that deserves to be called progressive, since it
> is progressive to see the psychoanalytic discourse founded, insofar as
> the latter completes the circle that could perhaps enable you to locate
> what it is exactly you are rebelling against—which doesn't stop that
> thing from continuing incredibly well.
>
> (pp. 207–208)

This encounter reflects Lacan's attempt to maintain a commitment to "the
truth about truth" (Lacan, 1986/1992, p. 184), namely, that the truth is only
ever half-said. What is repressed in the master's discourse and suppressed in
the consumerist discourse is that no one claiming the whole truth has more
than half of it.

Lacan's (1991/2007) reference to "complet[ing] the circle" is something
he brought up again in February the following year, a few months after this
confrontation. In his lecture on February 18, 1970, he noted that the master's discourse "embraces everything, even that which thinks of itself as
revolutionary, or more exactly as what is romantically called Revolution

with a capital R. The master's discourse accomplishes its own revolution in the other sense of doing a complete circle" (p. 87). "The sons kill the father," as André Green put it (Lacan, 1973/1978, p. 215). Revolution is constituted not by a true discursive transformation but by completing a circuit that begins and ends with the master's discourse—it's only a matter of which term occupies the place of S1.

None of this is to say that Lacan was reactionary (see Herron, 2016); it is to say that the use of psychoanalysis to buttress particular positions in the political field, while certainly conceivable, is a misuse of psychoanalysis and will ultimately shape psychoanalysis and the population of analysands who seek it in ways foreign to psychoanalysis itself.

I do not labor under the undoubtedly false impression that this essay will convince anyone not to deploy Lacan or psychoanalysis for political purposes; my much more modest hope is that it might degrade the alacrity with which we reach for Lacan or Freud to argue geopolitics, particularly when it comes to providing interpretations of the unconscious motivations of those who are not our analysands in contexts that are not analyses. It seems worth noting that Lacan's comments about being "anti-progressive" in the confrontation at Vincennes came in 1969, just after a period of remarkable polarization in 1968 (McCoy & Press, 2022). This polarization is not unlike today's, and it is interesting to note that Webster's (2022) take on Lacan's anti-progressiveness has to do with Lacan's unwillingness to buy into a historicist view of society, owing to the nonlinear nature of time. Perhaps it makes perfect sense for the psychoanalytic community—as would any community—to reach for its leaders for comfort in difficult times. Nonetheless, such reaching and such deployment of psychoanalytic theory seems rarely to lead to ethical outcomes.

The challenges of psychoanalysis are greater than merely navigating its own exigencies, however. If it is to have anything to say about the youth mental health crisis, it must find a way of engaging with a non-psychoanalytic society. With this in mind, how can psychoanalysis, a practice focused on the singular subject, approach a problem of desire—itself the consequence of a loss of initiation rites—at a social level while maintaining its "non-desire to cure" (Lacan, 1986/1992, p. 219)? This is that to which I will attend next.

Notes

1 This is an allusion to Lacan's (1977) words, "une pratique sans valeur" in the 24th year of his seminar, *L'insu que sait de l'une-bévue s'aile à mourre* (p. 156).
2 I do not believe this is the proper venue to go into detail over these matters as I could not possibly honor the situation adequately in the course of making a different argument. Nevertheless, I mention it here as a raw example of the susceptibility of psychoanalysis to polarization. For anyone reading this book who was not a member of an American psychoanalytic group in 2023, you can find more information in the article the Guardian published on the matter (Conroy, 2023).

References

Aristotle. (1907). *The poetics of Aristotle*. S. H. Butcher (Ed.). (S. H. Butcher, Trans.). MacMillan and Company. (Original work published ca. 335 BCE.)

Conroy, J. O. (2023, June 16). Inside the war tearing psychoanalysis apart. *The Guardian*. www.theguardian.com/education/2023/jun/16/george-washington-university-professor-antisemitism-palestine-dc.

Durkheim, E. (1997). *Suicide*. G. Simpson (Ed.). (J. A. Spaulding & G. Simpson, Trans.). Free Press. (Original work published 1897.)

Freud, S. (1930) Civilization and its discontents. *The Standard Edition of the Complete Psychological Works of Sigmund Freud* (Vol. XXI), pp. 57–146. Hogarth Press.

Freud, S. (1939) Moses and monotheism: Three essays. *The Standard Edition of the Complete Psychological Works of Sigmund Freud* (Vol. XXIII), pp. 1–138. Hogarth Press.

Herron, S. (2016). Reflecting on revolutions in France: Lacan and Burke. *Theory & Event*, 19(1). Project MUSE. muse.jhu.edu/article/607275.

Kant, I. (2004). *Critique of practical reason*. (T. K. Abbott, Trans.). Project Gutenberg. www.gutenberg.org/files/5683/5683-h/5683-h.htm (Original work published 1788.)

Lacan, J. (1977). 19 Avril 1977. *L'insu que sait de l'une-bévue s'aile à mourre*. Unpublished. www.valas.fr/IMG/pdf/S24_L_INSU—.pdf.

Lacan, J. (1978). *The four fundamental concepts of psychoanalysis*. J. A. Miller (Ed.). (A. Sheridan, Trans.). W.W. Norton & Co. (Original work published 1973.)

Lacan, J. (1992). *The Ethics of Psychoanalysis* (J. A. Miller, Ed., D. Porter, Trans.). W. W. Norton & Co. (Original work published 1986.)

Lacan, J. (1998). *On feminine sexuality, the limits of love and knowledge*. J. A. Miller (Ed.). (B. Fink, Trans.). W.W. Norton & Co. (Original work published 1975.)

McCoy, J. & Press, B. (2022). What happens when democracies become perniciously polarized?Carnegie Endowment for International Peace. https://carnegieendowment.org/2022/01/18/what-happens-when-democracies-become-perniciously-polarized.

Mueller, A. S., Abrutyn, S., Pescosolido, B., & Diefendorf, S. (2021). The social roots of suicide: Theorizing how the external social world matters to suicide and suicide prevention. *Frontiers in Psychology*, 12, 621569. doi:10.3389/fpsyg.2021.621569.

Nobus, D. (2016). Psychoanalytic violence: An essay on indifference in ethical matters. *Psychoanalytic Discourse*, 2, 1–20. https://psychoanalyticdiscourse.com/index.php/psyd/article/view/23/22.

Nobus, D. (2022). *Critique of psychoanalytic reason*. Routledge.

Soler, C. (2018). *Humanisation? Psychoanalysis, symbolisation, and the body of the unconscious*. (B. Farrow & H. D'Alascio, Trans.). Routledge.

Webster, J. (2022). *Disorganisation & Sex*. Divided Publishing.

12 Fantasia

Introduction

In 2002, when contemplating the wending trajectories of psychoanalysis in the 20th and early 21st centuries, Jacques-Alain Miller (2019) demarcated three periods of Lacan's work, divided less by chronology or evolution in theory as such than by the changes of society during these periods. The first period he characterized as one of disciplinary organization, where "there is a relation of exteriority between the apparatuses of repression and of training, on the one hand, and the subjugated on the other" (pp. 98–99). This era had the challenges of a real, physical oppression, but the benefit of having a clear exterior enemy to oppose at the same time.

The second era was "marked by the demedicalisation of the treatment," wherein the traversal of the fundamental fantasy came to the fore as an end of treatment (Miller, 2019, p. 101). This period was a transitional one between the disciplinary period of the Victorian era and the era of globalization, which itself characterizes the third period. Miller placed a second dictum alongside Lacan's "there is no sexual rapport," that "there is nothing but *jouissance*" (p. 103). This is in part a consequence of the "banalisation of the sexual spectacle today, from the pornographic film to Catherine Millet's latest book," a banalization all the more complete in the permeation of the smartphone, social media, and the corporatization of pornography (p. 94). The resultant damage is to the "social bond, which exists in the form of uprooted and dispersed subjects" (p. 124). There is no longer any (even fantasmatically) homogenous polity.

What makes Miller's (2019) reflections remarkable is not so much that they are novel at this point—his ideas about psychoanalysis and globalization, and similar ones alongside, are well-known today—but that they seem to silently fall along the lines of Fukuyama's (1992) end of history. This is not a criticism; any writing will show age after 20 years. But the change in sociopolitical landscape since then raises new issues to consider today in formulating psychoanalysis for a new time.

DOI: 10.4324/9781032666334-17

Interestingly, in the same lecture in 2002, at a moment when "the triumph of democracy…has the wind in its sails in the spirit of the time," Miller (2019) observed that:

> Totalitarianism was a great hope, it enchanted the masses of the twentieth century. In the twenty-first century, it is something that we barely recall. Totalitarianism was the hope of reabsorbing the division of truth, of establishing the reign of the One in the field of politics in accordance with the model of *Massenpsychologie*.
>
> (p. 88)

Totalitarianism, in Miller's reading, was a response to the fracturing of the world of polity. Miller related such fracturing to the break-up of what Lyotard called meta-narrative, resulting in a splintering of society such that totalitarianism would have a credible pull on the unconscious of so many. When the semblants one could previously rely upon begin to splinter, the totalitarian turn offers a way out.

While Miller's (2019) primary interest at the time of these remarks was the question of psychoanalysis in an increasingly globalized world, one is struck, from the perspective of the 2020s, with the degree to which his remarks about a time "we barely recall" actually bring forth recollections many in the US can now hardly forget (p. 88). In other words, the call of totalitarianism is echoing in the chambers of power once again. The notion of "reabsorbing the division of truth" remains tempting to all participants in discourse after consumerism (Miller, 2019, p. 88). It speaks to the power of the temptation to exclude anything unknown about oneself or the world; the division of truth, which isolates the truth as an inaccessible part of discourse and renders it only half-said, remains a target of reabsorption in today's imaginary and polarized society. This call toward authoritarianism is not an exclusively right-wing danger (Conway et al., 2021; Conway et al., 2023; Costello et al., 2022), although it is currently most present on the right-wing of the political spectrum in the US, which has a leader ready to answer the call. However, the diffuse listing toward authoritarianism on the left and its contrast with the authoritarian personality of the right echoes the distinction Guy Debord (1967/1983) drew between *diffuse* spectacle and *concentrated* spectacle; the irony, of course, being that the bureaucratic police state of concentrated spectacle was associated more with Maoist and Stalinist authoritarianism while the diffuse spectacle was more characteristic of American capitalism. This echo is only partial, however; the fact is that the authoritarianism of the right does seem increasingly consistent with concentrated spectacle while the left seems to move toward the integrated spectacle Debord (1988/1998) later interpolated into his theory. The integrated spectacle has no "known leader, or clear ideology," affects every part of life, and creates the reality it describes (p. 9). If the psychoanalysis of the past had a tendency toward concentrated spectacle, the field today—at least in the US—is susceptible to the integrated spectacle capable of enveloping any non-local community (i.e., one not built around physical proximity).

The totalitarianism of the 20th century was multifaceted but represented at least in part a struggle of national identifications and the identities of peoples in the face of increasing confrontation with difference within the body politic. The search for a unifying social relation in modern society is central to Debord's (1967/1983) spectacle, as it "presents itself...*as an instrument of unification*," but "the unification it achieves is nothing but an official language of generalized separation" (§ 3). The hypermodern search for unification seems to mirror this in an era of screens and the images that now constitute social life rather than represent it. The risk today is of a unifying message that actually only reifies separation; "the spectacle reunites the separate, but reunites it *as separate*" (§ 29). This separation should not be confused with the operation of separation in psychoanalysis; the latter is the condition of social relation while the former is the strangulation of it.

The question of totalitarianism is relevant because of its call and temptation. Only two years after Miller's (2019) previous comments, he gave a lecture at the fourth Congress of the World Association of Psychoanalysis titled "A Fantasy" (p. 139).[1] In considering a time after the Father in this lecture, Miller criticized those he called "Freudian fundamentalists," whom he argued wanted a return of the Father who could order things properly once again (p. 150). He likely had in mind, at least in part, the recent change in French law, which many psychoanalysts disputed, that no longer required children to bear their father's surname (Nobus, 2002). The protests of psychoanalysts in response certainly seem to mark a reactionary tendency. In addition to this, Miller (2019) identified a second line of response from analysts after the Father, while not a call for a second coming of the Father, no less problematic in its own way; Miller called this second response a nostalgic position which pretends there is no societal change occurring. The Father is still present, and everything may proceed as usual. Finally, he noted a third possibility of re-approaching psychoanalysis from a new paradigm just as Lacan came to Freud's psychoanalysis with a new paradigm (that of linguistics, initially). For example, psychoanalysis might move from a linguistic paradigm into neuropsychoanalysis, or a more cognitively or neurologically based paradigm. However, such a transmigration of psychoanalysis does not directly address the problem of initiation rites that is secondary to the changing of the Father's social standing.

Miller's (2019) reflection on Freudian fundamentalism hopefully gives more body to the ethical concerns of the last chapter. The most tempting resolution of the lack of initiation rites would be a certain recursion to the Father, one imposed as an external authority with all of the power and the glory of the imaginary Father. Psychoanalysts are not immune, under any circumstances, to the romance of the capital R Revolution (Lacan, 1991/2007). One must remember that the Father is not a person, and a puritanical adherence to doxa can constitute the master's discourse as well as any person. A psychoanalysis ready to champion political causes seems likely to find itself tearing down the very edifices upon which it is built.[2] If Miller (2019) could fantasize that the dominant discourse of society after the Father is the discourse of the analyst—a rather dubious assertion[3] one might feel grateful appeared in the context of a flight of fantasy—then one might conceivably fantasize that the "other side" of society, where the analyst positions themselves, is today the position of the master. Whether this is the case in other parts of the world is beyond the scope of this book, but U.S. psychoanalytic groups have shown a surprising penchant—in almost equal measures on the right and left—for a master's discourse that could set aright the problems of society, which have—according to both the right and left—infected psychoanalysis.

The most pertinent of the ideas Miller (2019) shared with respect to initiation rites is the way in which he placed sexual non-rapport at the center of the trouble in society today. The failure of the master's discourse—and particularly of master signifiers—means that "master signifiers no longer manage to give any existence to the sexual rapport" (p. 156). In Miller's account, civilization at the time of Freud was predicated on a certain arrangement between the individual and society, namely: "in order to give existence to the sexual relation, *jouissance* must be restrained, inhibited, repressed" (p. 157). This is a pithy Lacanian rendering of Freud's (1930) arrangement of society as a sublimation of some portion of the libido in exchange for fraternal and social relationships that make the social bond possible. Without the fantasy of a sexual rapport any longer, there is no easily available limit on *jouissance* and this is precisely why the panoply of solutions called the youth mental health crisis (suicide, self-injury, depression, identification with the stigma of diagnosis, and political polarization) are substitutionary, if not contrary, to the formation of the social link.

Miller's (2019) fantasy, or flight of fantasy, brings to mind the way in which these attempts by youth to resolve their entry to the social link operate as a sort of fantasia, in every sense of the term. They are improvisations, they contain elements that are already known but reorganized, and they may be surreal. As Svolos (2017) put it, after *the* Father has receded, the question for psychoanalysis becomes, "can we help those who come to see us for help to construct those signifiers—the names of the father—that have had a significatory—and significant—function in their lives?" (p. 35). This leads to a crucial question: What, in essence, is the crisis?

Nobus (2002) provided a rather pointed takedown of the view that the diminution of the Father is at the root of new social ills. I believe he correctly objected to the supposition that "new symptoms" are in fact new symptoms; holding open the possibility of changes in symptoms and subjectivities is, as discourse itself changes, reasonable (see Fink, 2017). However, I am more inclined to identify changes in "presenting concerns" as epiphenomenon or, if anything, changes in discourse that affect subjectivity without necessarily transmuting it, which is in line with Guerra's (2020) observation as well. At the same time, Nobus' (2002) skepticism about the significance of the diminution of the Father may have been overly compensatory for the conduct of francophone psychoanalysts at the time. The Father is more robust than this. I believe this to be the case not because the Father is somehow immutable but because humanity is much slower to change than many people appreciate, and the structure of the speaking being necessitates what Lacan called the Father. However, it is noteworthy that, as Svolos (2017) observed:

> By the end of Lacan's work, "mother" and "father" are less present. The notion of the master signifier, the sinthome, and even the notion of the One will, in the final work of Lacan, come to hold aspects of the function of the Name of the Father.
>
> (p. 33)

This is the same path Lacan followed in considering castration to be a result of language. The very structure of signification necessitates certain functions that cannot be done without—such as that executed by a master signifier. The changes to the legal familial structure of Western hypermodern societies portend changes neither in the structure of language itself nor in the fundaments of psychic structure. Because of this:

> To talk about the Name of the Father today, for us, is not linked to any kind of return to a mythically ideal time of the father, or, say, to any particular religious or ideological tradition. A task in psychoanalysis may be to identify what Names of the Father may be functioning in the discourse surrounding the child, as the discourses are structured in some way.
>
> (p. 34)

The soundness of this infrastructure is what necessitates the continued relevance of whatever one chooses to call the Father today.

Thus, the confidence Nobus cited in Federn's sentiment that the strength of the father is "deeply anchored in humanity through family education, and once again this will probably preclude the continuation of a completely 'fatherless society'" (as cited in Nobus, 2002, p. 185), although Federn's idea was undoubtedly more concrete.

Nobus' (2022) view that the enervation of the Father is not causative of new symptoms has some additional nuance worth considering. In particular, he identified the confusion of "the symbolic matrix with the social machinery" as the source of problematic entanglements of psychoanalysis in society (p. 188). As he put it:

> It is exactly because the social is confused with the symbolic that psychoanalysts believe they have the right (and the duty) to reflect upon the

deleterious impact of alternative kinship patterns on psychic health, and to discard them as pathogenic alterations.

(p. 188)

The social-symbolic confusion certainly underlies the Freudian fundamentalist position. The collapse of the imaginary and social, in turn, underlies another set of problematics within psychoanalysis.

At this point, it should be clear that the problem of initiation rites pertains not to actual paternity nor to the actual presence of a human father in the life of a child—though the presence or absence of such a figure and its articulation in the filial discourse no doubt has an impact on the child. Instead, the problem is as outlined in the preceding chapters with respect to the structural and symbolic function of the Father. In particular, the issue is that initiation rites do not today provide an articulation of the youth in discourse that connects them to a metanarrative, however tenuous it might be. As Kwame Anthony Appiah (2005) wrote:

> It matters to people that they can tell a story of their lives that meshes with larger narratives. This may involve rites of passage into womanhood and manhood; or a sense of national identity that fits one's life into a larger saga.
>
> (p. 68)

However, it is not only a matter of narrative, but in particular the way that narrative—or what Lacanians call fantasy—can structure suffering, or *jouissance*. Svolos (2017) wrote that "the meaning of suffering is not pre-determined…. The meaning is constructed by the patient, by the analyst, during the psychoanalytic experience" (p. 35). The narrative or meaning is not merely about attributing a sense of importance to the ego. It is a matter of constructing an identity within the Other that sustainably names *jouissance*. I would argue that, where Appiah uses narrative and Svolos uses meaning, it might be more precise to target within narrative and within meaning specifically the *nomination* that binds the registers together—the *sinthome*.

Lacan (2005/2016) observed that sexual non-rapport "must…assume some shape, and it does so not just any old how" (p. 56). In connection with this, he defined psychoanalysis as:

> The response to a riddle…. This is precisely why one must keep a firm hold on the rope. I mean that, if one has no idea where the rope ends, namely, in the knot of sexual non-relation, one runs the risk of floundering.
>
> (p. 57)

In this sense, psychoanalysis must do something with the sexual non-rapport against which the subject presses; without an initiation rite around the sexual development of puberty, this becomes all the more critical. Lacan identified the intervention of psychoanalysis with respect to this response to the riddle of non-rapport as a suture or splice. This is a somewhat different use of suture than Miller's (1966/1977) suture; it is the suture or splice of knot theory, wherein the Borromean link is sutured into an open trefoil knot (Lacan, 2005/2016, p. 58). In describing this, Lacan elaborated that:

> We really need to perform a suture somewhere between this symbolic, which stretches out here on its own, and this imaginary, which is here. It is a splice between the imaginary and unconscious knowledge. All of this is done to obtain a meaning, which is the object of the analyst's response to what the analysand exposes at length through his symptom.
>
> When we perform this splice, by the same stroke we make another one, precisely between that which is symbolic and the real. That is to say, in one way or another we teach the analysand to splice, to perform a splice between his sinthome and the parasitic real of jouissance. This is what typifies our operation. To make this jouissance possible is the same thing as what I shall write *j'ouïs-sens*. It is the same thing as *ouïr*, hearing, a *sens*, a meaning.
>
> (p. 58)

The *j'ouïs-sens* is crucial to the intervention that psychoanalysis can make regarding the state of things today for youth insofar as it characterizes the operation of splicing by artifice. Notably, where the splicing of which Lacan spoke is explicitly the splicing of registers within the subject, there is, today, a need for a splicing with respect to discourse. The parasitic real of *jouissance* is without a connecting point in the symbolic.

Thus, the failure of symbolic nomination makes all the more acute the need for the *sinthome*, which is not only an outcome for those with psychotic structures. The failure of nomination is the reason for the deployment of a nomination of disorder, assumed as stigmata, and the assumption of the imaginary as nomination in image-based polarizations. The question, in the end, is what can psychoanalysis offer, if anything, to this fantasia or variations on a theme of nomination?

Overall, there are two ways in which psychoanalysis has something to offer in the context of what is called the youth mental health crisis. One is proper to psychoanalysis, that is, to the practice of psychoanalysis as a clinical engagement, while the other is a riskier proposition: the use of psychoanalysis to inform public policy.

Psychoanalytically Informed Policy

It should by now be clear that I have a deep well of skepticism towards the deployment of psychoanalysis for political purposes. As Lacan (1991/2007) argued:

the intrusion into the political can only be made by recognizing that the only discourse there is, and not just analytic discourse, is the discourse of *jouissance*, at least when one is hoping for the work of truth from it.

(p. 78)

That is, any attempt to execute the work of Truth is always predicated on one's *jouissance*. This does not mean psychoanalysts do not have something to say, as citizens, about politics, but that psychoanalysis itself—as a body, a set of theories, an association of individuals identified by the particularity of being psychoanalytic, whatever this means—is in no way privileged to suppose it knows the Truth of social goods. Hecq (2006) summarized this by stating that "psychoanalysis does not purport to exert any power" (p. 217). Yet too often, however, psychoanalytic theory is a plowshare beaten into a sword, betraying the essence of the psychoanalytic position in order to engage in the ordering of social goods. This is the devolution of psychoanalysis into psychotherapy. This is also in-and-of-itself problematic for psychoanalysis to the extent that any attempt to order social goods addresses only ego identifications rather than subjectivity. Such interventions can only be particular, perhaps universal, and never singular.

Because of these many reasons for eschewing an intrusion into politics by psychoanalysis, it seems dubious to offer much in the way of a psychoanalytically informed policy. However, it is also the case that there is something to Lacan's (1967) statement that "the unconscious is politics" (p. 122). Miller (2019) interpreted this as an extension of Lacan's (1966/2006) "the unconscious is the Other's discourse," such that the Other is radically connected to subjectivity (p. 436). Lacan (1967) himself made this rather explicit, in another way, by clarifying his statement "the unconscious is politics," saying, "I mean that what binds men together, or what opposes them, is precisely to be justified by that whose logic we are trying for the moment to articulate," that is, the logic of fantasy (p. 122). If there is an intervention to be made in a psychoanalytic fashion at the level of policy, it can only be something that intervenes at the level of an artifice of fantasy that enables the subject to splice, in some fashion, the parasitic real of *jouissance*.

Given that the discourse of consumerism that lies at the root of the twilight of the civil religion and the increasingly insidious use of technology, attempts to put the toothpaste back in the bottle with respect to sexual knowledge are entirely misguided. This is not to advocate for the total removal of guardrails with respect to sexuality for youth—and the Internet sorely needs more such guardrails—but such guardrails only go halfway, and they do not address the actual dual problem of identification and integration that create any ground for a prohibition.

There is only one version of policy that I could imagine might provide an intervention at the level of fantasy and structure, such that splicing might become more feasible for youth. Such a policy would be a truly nationwide engagement from youth pertinent to the national community itself. Mandatory national service is the only such engagement that could accomplish something like this. Importantly, this is a relatively non-partisan issue, and one a surprisingly large number of people support (Cohen, 2023; see also Brooks, 2020; Mason & Liu, 2019). Also important is that such mandatory service should not entail mandatory military service. One outline of such a program is as follows:

> All citizens and permanent residents (Green Card holders) will be required to participate in an 18-month National Service program. Service can be started any time between an individual's 18th [and] 22nd birthday. Service shall include healthcare assistance, infrastructure/environmental repair, early childhood education programs, eldercare assistance, or military service. Participation in the military option shall be voluntary. National service participants shall receive free communal room, board, and a subsistence allowance. Participants shall receive $10,000 upon successful completion of their service. People who fail to successfully complete their National Service obligation shall not be eligible for any Federal student loan or mortgage guarantee program.
>
> (Cohen, 2023, para. 4)

This sort of program would allow for a significant variety in what young persons would actually do in the process of their service.

While it is not new to suggest that such a service could help heal political polarization in the country (Mason & Liu, 2019), I am not aware of any literature connecting such service directly to youth mental health. It is not simply exposure to others different than oneself that would make a difference, although this would certainly be part of the benefit. Rather, the most stratospheric impact would be the elevation, in a consumerist and hedonist society, of an act of service. While teenage years are often portrayed in the national consciousness as a time of partying and rambunctious shenanigans—most painfully bound up with the injunction to enjoy—the introduction of a mandatory service would provide both a real initiation into adulthood as well as an identification of something that one can point to as constituting an "American" (in the U.S. sense).

One may reasonably inquire what information about the sexual relation something like mandatory national service could dream of imparting. Insofar as the mandatory nature of the service places a limit on *jouissance*, it would create the conditions from which, in Freudian-Lacanian terms, the fantasy of rapport would spring forth. The fantasy is a response to the condition of desire, which is the limit of *jouissance*, and creating these conditions would inevitably create the illusion of the sexual rapport if for no other reason than for the belief that one had done some good in their service and the hope that they could, in fact, return home again.

Obviously, this is in itself a significant ethical proposal, one that would limit the free will of youth to some degree. This is properly a feature rather than a bug, as the interdiction is precisely what is needed for the limitation of *jouissance* in desire. Nonetheless, I must again note that despite describing this in psychoanalytic terms—terms I find compelling—it is not thereby a psychoanalytic proposal.

One motivating factor for considering such a sweeping proposal is that the alternative may be much more costly and concerning. The toll of polarization and the loss of unifying narratives has resulted in a volatile situation in which civil war is no longer unthinkable (Ottesen, 2022; Simon & Stevenson, 2023). The non-partisan Public Religion Research Institute found in a 2023 survey that 38 percent of Americans would support authoritarianism and almost a quarter believe political violence may be necessary to restore the nation. Such civil conflict would likely not be as structured as the previous U.S. Civil War, with conflict spread within states and in smaller sectarian violence (Bonenberger, 2023; Elving, 2022).

The current tinderbox of U.S. politics suggests that perhaps society has not ultimately changed as significantly as those predicting the end of the Father have supposed. It remains to be seen how long society will permit the Father to stay dead. After all, the Father is alive and well in Russia and the People's Republic of China and is growing more vital in other nations. The speaking being cannot, at bottom, exist without the necessary exception ($\exists x \bar{\Phi} \bar{x}$) and there will always be a pull for an order privileging this exception, whether the language of the Father is retained or abandoned in favor of something less historically freighted. In one form or another, there will be a second coming.

One might certainly envision other forms of psychoanalytically informed action that could address the youth mental health crisis in some way. These would almost invariably, in my view, entail far more dubious propositions than even something as ambitious as mandatory national service. For example, one might propose opening a series of Freudian-Lacanian clinics to treat youth; this seems like a quixotic proposal as it relies on too few analysts serving too many people, many of whom likely have a skepticism and reticence towards psychoanalysis thanks to the U.S. educational system. Moreover, any intervention targeting a particular group rather than a universal structure seems likely to privilege certain characteristics in a form of moral judgment. That is to say, supposing there was a Freudian-Lacanian intervention that was able to serve some subset of youth, how would it be decided which youth would receive this intervention? It would almost invariably have to be based on some characteristic of the youth's individual or their circumstances, but in no case on their subjectivity, and such a judgment of circumstances would require the determination that an individual is lacking in some fashion—morally—compared to another. Even so, perhaps someone will come up with an idea that does not fall into one of these traps (the impossible and the moralistic).[4]

Clinical Psychoanalytic Work

The response of psychoanalysis is most appropriate, of course, at the clinical level. In this case, there is no universal technique of intervention, nor I do not intend to provide a comprehensive taxonomy of technical skills, but rather to offer certain illustrative observations that may help to guide clinical work in some fashion. One preliminary note is that Lacanian psychoanalysis is uniquely positioned to contribute to the treatment of youth today, especially compared to skills-based therapies. While these help in some cases, until such a time as youth begin to integrate more fully into the social link (with the regulation attendant to it), psychoanalysis will be of increased importance for youth.

The presentation of the types of youth described in the previous chapters gives some idea of what the clinic of the mental health crisis may look like. Notably, those who find in political polarization a substitute for the social bond may not present to treatment—or if they do, only for help with learning skills to advocate for changing their environments. There is not a symptom in such cases apart from civilization. Despite the fact that suffering still may exist here, these are not cases wherein it is likely that a psychoanalytic treatment will produce results; this is not what such youth are looking for. In some ways, polarization—particularly how it places one into an ideological frame in social media—is similar to Miller's (2019) interpretation of the *otaku* as one who restricts their interests to "limited zones of certitude" (p. 123). This is problematic from the perspective of the social link, but for a psychoanalysis with an ethic of a non-desire to cure, this is not something to be helped.

In contrast, the youth most in subjective distress seem to be those in the first group, discussed in Chapter 7, experiencing as they are suicidal thoughts, non-suicidal self-injury, and severe depression that are difficult to extract from the familial and societal environments from which they grow. In my view, the difficulties encountered by these youth are the end product of a long chain of issues, stretching from the social link's previous decay that has left the parents without adequate integration and regulation, which has in turn led the parents to use the child as symptom or a "correlate of a fantasy," that is, as an object of *jouissance* (Lacan, 1986/2018). This in turn leads to the problems of acting out that can characterize these youth (Waitz, 2022).

Several things make clinical work with youth today somewhat different compared to such work in the past or work with adults, although this does not call for wild innovation in theory as long as one has a correct understanding of the situation. Certain aspects of treatment are simply more important or look slightly different in the clinic of uninitiated youth. For example, when working with patients experiencing symptoms related to a lack of initiation, it is of increased importance to maintain a separate role from any other adult in the youth's life, a role predicated not on the enforcement of anything—and certainly not on the enforcement of the happiness parents and systems often demand. This is less a technical recommendation and more an observation of the importance of the analyst's desire. Other important aspects of this work are the inclusion, in some cases, of the parents in a more active way, the willingness on the part of the clinician to entertain a certain directiveness in using the transference (within the confines Lacan [1966/2006] outlined), and the way in which the facilitation of an identification is central—not an identification with the analyst, but with something capable of sustaining a social bond. The facilitation of an identification is neither an ethical imperative nor a developmentalist intervention, but a response to the demand of the child in the session when reading the message to the Other contained in acting out. The facilitation of this identification must be in the form of the splice, that which, in *j'ouïs-sens*, provokes in the youth a response of making a narrative of their suffering that splices, through the *sinthome*, the real, imaginary, and symbolic, in particular in such a way that delimits *jouissance*.

In an example I wrote about in 2022, I described how the use of directives given to a young person's mother might result in the creation of a space for desire between the mother and child. Such directives included instructions to write questions regarding the child's language in session, specifically writing only questions to which the mother did not know the answer. Having the mother articulate these questions at the end of each session, and ending with these questions unanswered, began to create space in the mother's mind for something other than demand. By utilizing a degree of direction in this work, the subject's circuit of desire began to become established in a reciprocal questioning—*what do you want?*—that necessarily enlivens fantasy and begins to confront the subject with something other than the Other's use of them. In this case, the youth's suicidal behaviors, including suicide attempts, were, in the course of the work, articulated as acting out in the sense of constituting a message to the Other (Lacan, 1998/2017). This provided a splice of the parasitic real to the symbolic, generating an ability for the youth to begin to identify with something other than the *jouissance* of the Other.

In another case, I worked with a 12-year-old boy in a residential setting who was frequently hospitalized for aggression. This child's symptom, however, was hallucinatory visions of a demon who would command aggressive acts. The process of our clinical work largely revolved around an unfolding of the parental relationship under which this young subject fell sway. When he was young, his mother had, for understandable reasons, created some barriers between the child and his father, yet he did not understand why these barriers were erected, particularly as his father was regularly part of his life again at the time I saw him. In working with this child, he began to articulate certain matters—having "too many" memories of his mother, a dream of her murder, feeling sad about his father's absence, and the presence of the demon, who happened to bear his father's name. In beginning to stitch connections between the imaginary demon, his father, and the function of separation that never fully occurred, this young person began to experience fewer outbursts of aggression. Interestingly, perhaps in part from directive instructions in sessions with his parents (e.g. instructing everyone where to sit in relation to one another), the mother came to articulate at the end of treatment that she had grown to use her child as, in her language, "a crutch."

Both of these cases are illustrative of what clinical work in the youth mental health crisis may entail. Owing to the nature of my work in institutions, my interventions are often at the level of crisis, after which point patients move to lower levels of care. In both cases, the work of true splicing largely lay ahead. However, by creating space for desire, for something outside the hedonistic *jouissance* of the now, each youth would have the opportunity to identify with something other than the object of *jouissance*. This is a way of, in Lacan's (2005/2016) words, coming to the point of there being "no jouissance of this Other of the Other" (p. 58). In the latter case, the 12-year-old had a tenuous relationship with their father that started to become strengthened in the course of our work. Although the actual father need not be the vehicle of identification that facilitates the departure from the insularity of the Oedipal triad (mother, child, phallus; Lacan, 1994/2020), it certainly can be.

With respect to the assumption of a diagnosis (as stigmata), this is an especially challenging area for intervention, as youth often do not have an interest in giving up their symptom (in the sense of descriptive psychiatry) when they present to treatment; instead, they want a nomination in the form of a diagnosis. Presenting with self-diagnosed dissociative identity disorder (which speaks to the fractures in the social link), autism (speaking to the outsideness of the subject with respect to the social link), borderline personality disorder (speaking to the importance of binding *jouissance* to a not-me clinical entity), or bipolar disorder (speaking to the use of biology in protecting one's symptom) are all common. What becomes important in these cases, as noted before, is the ability to maintain ambiguity, neither refusing the demand nor acceding to it. By creating space for curiosity, one can give the youth the opportunity to begin to articulate the exigencies of their desire for a diagnosis—again, ultimately creating the opportunity for there to be a splicing of the imaginary, symbolic, and real in discourse. Not all youth are up for this task, and some will decline to take it up. For those that are able, it can lead to a fruitful engagement around what is, in many cases, a significant matter of alienation as one has not been invited into the social link.

Working with uninitiated youth requires one to have one's bearings. Miller (2019) noted the way in which the capitalist discourse comes to privilege "the subject without bearings" (p. 126), so to find one's bearings is not a small feat. Without a sense of the new problematics appearing for youth today, it would become easy to get lost in the performances of acting out and the captures of fantasmatic identification that trouble the psyche and, in common sense approaches to psychotherapy, privilege the perpetuation of these rather than their resolution according to the demands of the youth involved.

Conclusion

The youth mental health crisis, in the sense of public health, is a problem of descriptive symptoms. The aggregation of these symptoms in ever greater numbers is the marker of crisis, and presumably the suffering indexed by these descriptive symptoms is of concern. The problem, then, is how to prevent as many youth as possible from experiencing the markers of distress and suffering, in general by improving their mental health. However, this improvement of mental health is often pegged, in terms of clinical intervention, to "coping" or emotion regulation, capacities which are taught through the delivery of a knowledge (*connaissance*) by a technician to a client. This is a largely mechanical conception of the person, wherein, as in automobile repair, the expert might replace a faulty part in the object in order to make things work. However, it is that which doesn't work that primarily interests psychoanalysis.

The labor of excavating the causes of a mental health crisis in "real time" is incredibly challenging for the tools of empirical science, and certainly not easier for psychoanalysis. That is, rightly dividing such complex societal forces and their effects is perhaps too ambitious a course, yet such work is vital to developing an understanding of how to respond to such societal changes.

In considering the youth mental health crisis in the early 21st century, I have argued that there are several interlocking issues involved, the confluence of which has effected the crisis. Durkheim's (1897/1997) *Suicide* offers an important resource for understanding the social link as comprising integration and regulation, two principles at the heart of Lacan's adoption of the social link (Miller & Vanheule, 2023). The principles of integration and regulation can be understood in Freudian-Lacanian terms as identification with the ego ideal and the prohibition of *jouissance*, respectively. The Name/No of the Father is the element that historically has navigated this dual function, which has precipitated the initiation rite as a transition from childhood to adulthood.

The Name of the Father has become eroded, owing to the forces of consumer capitalism, which has erased the role of truth as half-said and denies desire, as all desires must be fulfilled—thereby reducing them to demand. This has resulted in a rejection of the prohibition to increase profit. At the same time, civil religion has ceased to hold the political body of the US together in one identification, leading to factionalism across the board. Technology has only contributed to the acceleration of these forces, with social media simultaneously exposing youth to the absence of any metanarrative or semblant and providing sexual knowledge that excludes prohibition. The imaginary power of social media also contributes to privileging the ideal ego over against any other identification. Political polarization is a result of these problems and, at the same time, exacerbates them.

With the failure of initiation rites, these forces have led to decreasing numbers of youth successfully integrating in the social link and undergoing regulation of *jouissance*, such that youth have had to improvise extempore solutions. Such solutions include suicidal thoughts and behaviors, self-injury, and depression; identification through the nomination of a diagnosis; and succumbing to political polarization in order to develop a limited zone of certitude.

To address these concerns, there are a handful of options. The most grand would be—not a psychoanalytic solution—the introduction of a mandate for national service. The risk of political violence without some form of addressing the absence of the Name of the Father as organizing the social structure remains present. In clinical work, this may require special innovation and attempts to facilitate identification for the youth—a task of facilitation with which psychoanalytic clinicians may not naturally engage.

My hope in articulating this argument in such a manner is that it will become possible for others to begin to think and act in new ways in the face of what seems, at the surface, to be a changing environment of youth mental health care. In reality, while there are changes afoot, it remains to be seen how lasting such changes are.

Notes

1 The translators note that the French Une Fantasie is better rendered as something like "a flight of fantasy" (Miller, 2019, p. 139).
2 One might perhaps make an exception for agitation regarding regulatory decisions directly impacting the practice of psychoanalysis; for example, the efforts of Jacques Alain-Miller, Elisabeth Roudinesco, and others in working to limit state intervention in psychoanalysis (Cultures en mouvement, 2004).
3 This marks a point of agreement between Žižek (2006) and me.
4 Svolos's (2017) perspective on politics would likely class what I have laid out here as a symbolic policy, and rightfully so, in the sense that symbolic politics for Svolos are universal. I also believe Svolos is correct in highlighting the dangers of imaginary politics, which he relates to Nazism's fixation on racial identity. In frequent Lacanian style, Svolos served up these imaginary and symbolic politics as foils to what he would then suggest as a politics of the real. It is unclear what the practical consequences of his real politics would be, however. He mentions the *sinthome* and fashion, for example, but it is not really clear how a focus on singularity alone would organize the social link.

References

Appiah, K. A. (2005). *The ethics of identity*. Princeton Classics.
Bonenberger, A. (2023, December 24). A second American civil war wouldn't look like a movie. *The Hill*. https://thehill.com/opinion/national-security/4374348-a-second-american-civil-war-wouldnt-look-like-a-movie.

Brooks, D. (2020, May 7). We need national service. Now. *The New York Times*. www.nytimes.com/2020/05/07/opinion/national-service-americorps-coronavirus.html.

Cohen, S. (2023, October 15). Americans support mandatory national service. *The Hill*. https://thehill.com/opinion/campaign/4253664-americans-support-mandatory-national-service.

Conway, L. G., III, McFarland, J. D., Costello, T. H., & Lilienfeld, S. O. (2021). The curious case of left-wing authoritarianism: When authoritarian persons meet anti-authoritarian norms. *Journal of Theoretical Social Psychology*, 5(4), 423–442. doi:10.1002/jts5.108.

Conway, L. G., III, Zubrod, A., Chan, L., McFarland, J. D., & Van de Vliert, E. (2023). Is the myth of left-wing authoritarianism itself a myth? *Frontiers in Psychology*, 13, 1041391–1041391. doi:10.3389/fpsyg.2022.1041391.

Costello, T. H., Bowes, S. M., Stevens, S. T., Waldman, I. D., Tasimi, A., & Lilienfeld, S. O. (2022). Clarifying the structure and nature of left-wing authoritarianism. *Journal of Personality and Social Psychology*, 122(1), 135–170. doi:10.1037/pspp0000341.

Cultures en mouvement. (2004). A law regulating psychoanalysis in France: An historic turning point for psychoanalysis. (M. S. Lieberman, Trans.). *European Journal of Psychoanalysis*, 18. www.journal-psychoanalysis.eu/articles/a-law-regulating-psychoanalysis-in-france-an-historic-turning-point-for-psychoanalysis-1.

Debord, G. (1983). *Society of the spectacle*. Black & Red. (Original work published 1967.)

Debord, G. (1998). *Comments on the society of the spectacle*. (M. Imrie, Trans.). Verso. (Original work published 1988.)

Durkheim, E. (1997). *Suicide*. G. Simpson (Ed.). (J. A. Spaulding & G. Simpson, Trans.). Free Press. (Original work published 1897.)

Elving, R. (2022, January 11). Imagine another American Civil War, but this time in every state. *NPR*. www.npr.org/2022/01/11/1071082955/imagine-another-american-civil-war-but-this-time-in-every-state.

Fink, B. (2017). *A clinical introduction to Freud: Techniques for everyday practice*. W.W. Norton & Co.

Fukuyama, F. (1992). *The end of history and the last man*. Free Press.

Guerra, A. M. C. (2020). La nominación en la adolescencia. *Affectio Societatis (Medellín)*, 17(33), 112–132. doi:10.17533/udea.affs.v17n33a05.

Hecq, D. (2006). The impossible power of psychoanalysis. In J. Clemens & R. Grigg (Eds), *Jacques Lacan and the other side of psychoanalysis: Reflections on seminar XVII*, pp. 216–226. Duke University Press.

Lacan, J. (1967). *The logic of phantasy*. (C. Gallagher, Trans.). Unpublished seminar.

Lacan, J. (2006). *Ecrits*. (B. Fink, Trans.). W.W. Norton & Co. (Original work published 1966.)

Lacan, J. (2007). *The other side of psychoanalysis*. J. A. Miller (Ed.). (R. Grigg, Trans.). W.W. Norton & Co. (Original work published 1991.)

Lacan, J. (2016). *The sinthome*. J. A. Miller (Ed.). (A. R. Price, Trans.). Polity. (Original work published 2005.)

Lacan, J. (2017). *Formations of the Unconscious*. J. A. Miller (Ed.). (R. Grigg, Trans.). Polity. (Original work published 1998.)

Lacan, J. (2018). Note on the child. *The Lacanian Review*, 4, 13–14. (Original work published 1986.) https://lacancircle.com.au/wp-content/uploads/2018/04/Note-on-the-Child.pdf.

Lacan, J. (2020). *The object relation: The seminar of Jacques Lacan, Book* IV. J. A. Miller (Ed.). (A. R. Price, Trans.). Polity Press. (Original work published 1994.)

Mason, L. & Liu, E. (2019). Mandatory national service. *Politico.* www.politico.com/interactives/2019/how-to-fix-politics-in-america/polarization/mandatory-national-service.

Miller, A. & Vanheule, S. (2023). What Holds You Together: 'The Social Link' in Durkheim, Saussure and Lacan. *Psychoanalysis and History*, 25(1), 5–29. doi:10.3366/pah.2023.0450.

Miller, J. A. (1977). Suture. (J. Rose, Trans.). *Screen*, 18(4), 24–34. (Original work published 1966.)

Miller, J. A. (2019). *Paradigms of jouissance: Three interventions by Jacques-Alain Miller.* (T. Sowley, M. Julien, J. Haney, & A. Duncan, Trans.). Psychoanalytical Notebooks.

Nobus, D. (2002). Symptom and society: A clinical challenge for contemporary psychoanalysis. *Modern Psychoanalysis*, 27(2), 179–203.

Ottesen, K. K. (2022, March 8). 'They are preparing for war': An expert on civil wars discusses where political extremists are taking this country. *The Washington Post.* www.washingtonpost.com/magazine/2022/03/08/they-are-preparing-war-an-expert-civil-wars-discusses-where-political-extremists-are-taking-this-country.

Public Religion Research Institute. (2023). Threats to American democracy ahead of an unprecedented presidential election [White Paper]. www.prri.org/wp-content/uploads/2023/10/PRRI-Oct-2023-AVS.pdf.

Simon, S. & Stevenson, J. (2023, April 21). The threat of civil breakdown is real. *Politico.* www.politico.com/news/magazine/2023/04/21/political-violence-2024-magazine-00093028.

Svolos, T. (2017). *Twenty-first century psychoanalysis.* Karnac.

Waitz, C. (2022). Acting out and psychoanalytically informed treatment in inpatient adolescent psychiatry. *Psychoanalytic Psychology*, 39(3), 209–216. doi:10.1037/pap0000405.

Žižek, S. (2006). Jacques Lacan's four discourses. www.lacan.com/zizfour.htm.

Index

Note: locators followed by 'n' refer to notes.